Essential Oils
for *the* Whole Body

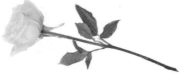

". . . offers a beautiful bridge between the science of aromatherapy and esoteric application. Godfrey presents a truly holistic approach that explores how to support the whole self, from the physical to the emotional and spiritual."

CANDICE COVINGTON, CERTIFIED AROMATHERAPIST, AUTHOR OF *ESSENTIAL OILS IN SPIRITUAL PRACTICE*, AND OWNER OF DIVINE ARCHETYPES

"A lovely book packed full of information about the form and function of the human body and the ways essential oils can interact with it. This book builds on the author's previous work, *Essential Oils for Mindfulness and Meditation,* to create an invaluable guide for those who wish to understand essential oils and use them creatively and safely."

SOPHIE OLSZOWSKI, PHD, DIRECTOR OF SPZ ASSOCIATES LTD.

"In times when most aromatherapists are going back to using simple recipes based on the biomedical paradigm, this book opens up another way of looking at topical applications and absorption dynamics. These areas are actually more complex than mechanical interpretation allows and require a book with a holistic, and even spiritual, background combined with scientific insight. It will surely build stronger relationships with the 'whole body.'"

MARTIN HENGLEIN, NATUROPATH, AROMATHERAPIST, AND OSMOLOGIST

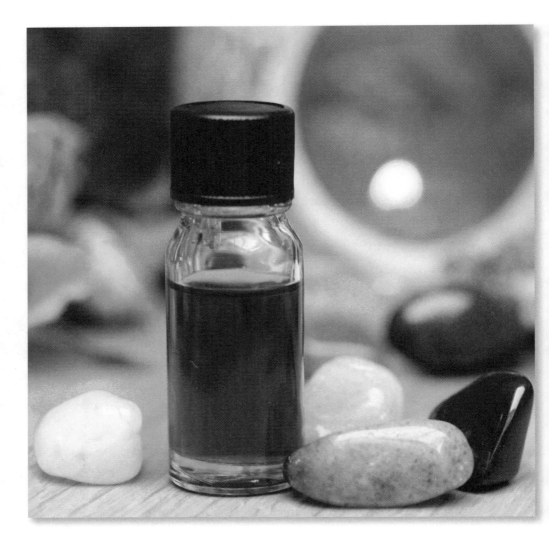

Essential Oils
for the Whole Body

The Dynamics of
Topical Application
and Absorption

Heather Dawn Godfrey, PGCE, BSc

Healing Arts Press
Rochester, Vermont

Healing Arts Press
One Park Street
Rochester, Vermont 05767
www.HealingArtsPress.com

Healing Arts Press is a division of Inner Traditions International

Note to the reader: This book is intended as an informational guide. The remedies, approaches, and techniques described herein are meant to supplement, and not to be a substitute for, professional medical care or treatment. They should not be used to treat a serious ailment without prior consultation with a qualified health care professional.

Cataloging-in-Publication Data for this title is available from the Library of Congress

ISBN 978-1-62055-871-3 (print)
ISBN 978-1-62055-872-0 (ebook)

Printed and bound in the United States by Versa Press, Inc.

10   9   8   7   6   5   4   3   2   1

Text design and layout by Virginia Scott Bowman
This book was typeset in Garamond Premier Pro, Gill Sans, and Frutiger with Modern used as the display typeface.

Illustration credits: page 8 by Genome Research Limited (www.yourgenome.org /facts/what-is-a-cell); pages 24, 27, 45, and 46 by W. Dowell and D. Smith, www .coastlinecreative.co.uk, 2017; page 25 by Patrick J. Lynch, medical illustrator (CC BY 2.5); page 182 by Murray Fagg (CC BY 3.0); page 188 by T. Voekler (CC BY-SA 3.0); page 196 by Lazaregagnidze (CC BY-SA 3.0); page 203 cropped from *Köhler's Medizinal-Pflanzen* illustration, courtesy of the Biodiversity Heritage Library (CC BY 2.0); page 206 from lovepik.com; page 214 by Marco Bernardini (CC BY-SA 3.0); page 217 by Forest & Kim Starr, http://starrenvironmental.com (CC BY 3.0); page 220 by Zeynel Cebeci (CC BY-SA 4.0); page 223 by H. Zell (GNU Free Documentation License); page 228 by Steven2 (Wikiwel); page 231 by Csubbra (CC BY-SA 3.0); page 234 by treesftf (CC BY 2.0)

To send correspondence to the author of this book, mail a first-class letter to the author c/o Inner Traditions • Bear & Company, One Park Street, Rochester, VT 05767, and we will forward the communication, or contact the author directly at **www.aromantique.co.uk**.

To my children,
Aaron, Sonny, April, and Leon,
my blessing and my teachers.

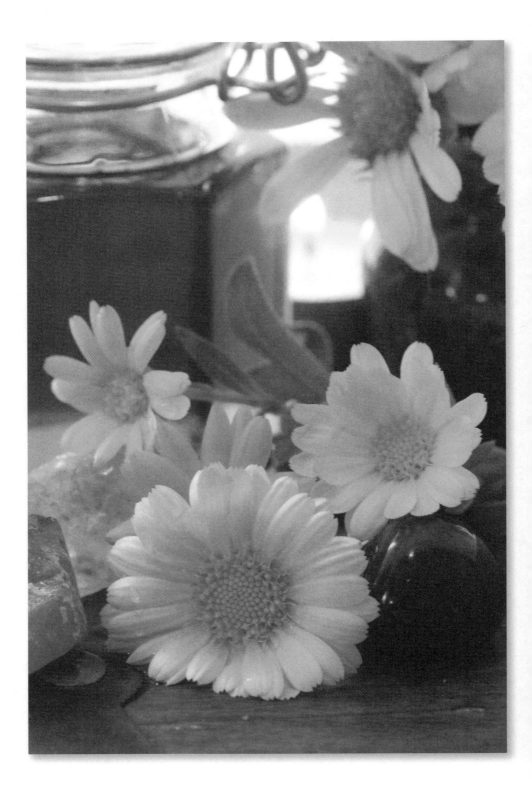

Contents

Preface

Complementary medicine has come a long way since I was first introduced to it in the early 1970s. In those days, "alternative" medicine, as it was known, was generally dismissed by the medical community as a hippie or fringe philosophy. Today, however, complementary medicine has come into its own as a proven, science-supported, intensively studied, and well-documented healing modality, and I remain eternally grateful that I became aware of it as I stepped out into the world as a curious teenager.

Meditation, in particular, was my saving grace as I traversed life's meandering path through the ups and downs and plateaus that present themselves on any journey. Though it is by no means a magic wand that instantly transports you to your "happy ever after," it grounded me when I felt adrift, gave inspiration when I lacked it, and renewed me when I felt depleted. The experience of meditation lent me great appreciation for the subtle tenets that underpin many ancient healing systems, such as the existence of vital energy—élan vital, prana, chi, life force, or whatever you would like to call it—even if it is difficult to explain to people who demand tangible physical evidence as proof.

Today, through the advancement of technologies, we are (re)discovering amazing insights about how the world works, about the body's incredible capacity to heal and self-regulate, and, significantly, about the resonant omnipresence and influence of vital energy, which permeates everything from the atom to all that is manifest in the world and universe (thanks to Albert Einstein, Stephen Hawking, and many others for their pioneering research). These insights verify and uphold the foundational dynamics established by the world's ancient healing modalities.

According to quantum physics, the invisible, immaterial realm has far more influence over us than the material realm; space, in fact, is not empty but alive with energy. Epigenetic research demonstrates that our conscious thoughts, unconscious beliefs, and emotions shape our biological development. That is, our internal response to our environment regulates our genetic expression. Neuroplastic research confirms that our brains are constantly being shaped and reshaped by our experiences. The structure and organization of the brain changes as we experience, learn, and adapt, and our neural pathways are reinforced by repetitive thoughts, attitudes, and actions. In this sense, we literally become the manifestation of what we think and do. It is an incredibly empowering realization.

What if there was a way to intentionally guide our internal response and thus make manifest positive changes we wish to realize in our bodies, psyches, and spirits? In fact, that is the subject of this book: using essential oils, which have uniquely powerful and holistic interactions with the human body, to benefit us physiologically, psycho-emotionally, and spiritually.

Everything in the universe, material or immaterial, resonates, or vibrates, including our thoughts. In a state of healthy function, the whole body resonates at a collective average electromagnetic wave or vibrational frequency of between 62 and 90 MHz; at this frequency the body is able to maintain resilience to disease and optimum health and wellness. American scientist and inventor Royal Rife (1888–1971) was an early proponent of the idea that vibrational frequencies had direct connections to our health. According to Rife, an average vibrational frequency below 61 MHz sees the body's resilience weaken and the immune system compromised, rendering it susceptible to disease, viral invasion, and chronic illness. Disease starts at 58 MHz; the body is vulnerable to cancer at 42 MHz. The higher our resonant frequency, therefore, the healthier, more resilient, and able to recover from trauma we are.

The body's vibrational frequency is positively influenced by many factors, such as the quality and substance of our food. Good-quality, nutritionally rich, organic food raises our vibrational frequency. Processed and canned foods, however, have *no* vibrational input. Laughter, happiness, positive thoughts and attitude, good-quality sleep, relaxation, meditation, yoga, and exercise also increase and sustain the body's vibrational frequency. The clarity of thought, mental alertness, positive mood, and good energy levels that result from these positive lifestyle choices are indicators of not just our body's state of health but also our vibrational frequency.

Like foods, which have nutritional components that we can isolate, identify, and measure, essential oils have chemical constituents that we can isolate, identify, and measure and that have measurable effects on human physiology. Good-quality essential oils are valued not just for their wonderful aromatics but also for their antimicrobial, immune-supportive, and restorative actions. We know that essential oils' molecules, when inhaled, trigger powerful effects in the brain, particularly in relation to the limbic system. We know that essential oils bring a host of healing benefits to the skin, and also that they readily penetrate the skin, bringing those benefits to the entire body via the circulatory system. But also like foods, essential oils bring a positive resonant frequency to the body. They elevate us, not just physically but vibrationally. They have a multidynamic effect on the body.

Through my practice, I have observed that essential oils are incredibly potent. Even very small amounts of essential oils procure meaningful physiological and psycho-emotional responses. In this book, we'll explore those responses and the very wide spectrum of essential oil qualities, from their very basic actions and scents to their interplay with the subtle energies of colors, gemstones, and chakras, all in the service of supporting, maintaining, and restoring our well-being.

My hope is that readers will come away from this book with a deeper appreciation for and understanding of the multisensory, multidynamic actions and energies of essential oils, and with a foundational knowledge of how to apply essential oils for holistic health—in body, mind, and spirit.

Happy journeys!

Her face shone with all the colors of a diamond in sunlight as they wooshed over the Rainbow Bridge. This bridge straddled space between silvery-blue Uranus and the darkness of Saturn. This was the gateway to a peaceful resting place before the final journey back to earth because, surely, by now, she had been away long enough. Here, it was like inside a kaleidoscope. There were so many colors and patterns, all very strong yet gentle at the same time. There were wonderful fragrances too. It was like walking through a perfume shop or scented garden. Issie sensed loving presences, though she saw no one. . . . It seemed as though these presences had been hurt themselves, so they knew how it felt to be wounded. They had learned how to heal themselves, so they could teach others.

CAROLINE MAYALL,
SUNSHINE AND MOONBEAMS STORIES

Acknowledgments

My sincere thanks and gratitude are extended, as always, to my daughter, April Sandrene Tatlock; to my godmother, May Copp; to my brother, Stephen Godfrey; to Pamela Allsop; and to Sophie Olszowski, for their unconditional support, belief, and encouragement. I also wish to thank my students and clients, past and present, for the privilege of working with them and for everything they continue teach me. And of course, I'd like to thank the Inner Traditions team for their professional support and diligence in producing this book from manuscript to printed page.

Many of the photographs featured in this book were taken with kind permission at Compton Acres, beautiful gardens spread over ten acres in Poole, England. My thanks and appreciation are extended to Joseph Coogan, gardener, for sharing his wealth of knowledge and expertise, and to Bernard Merna, owner of the gardens, for allowing me access, often before the gardens were open in the morning, to take the photographs.

The essential oils and vegetable oils featured in some of the photographs in this book were supplied by NHR Organic Oils (Brighton, Sussex, UK), Oshadhi (Cambridge, UK), Tisserand Aromatherapy (West Sussex, UK), the Frankincense Store (London, UK), and Base Formula Limited (Melton Mowbray, Leicestershire, UK).

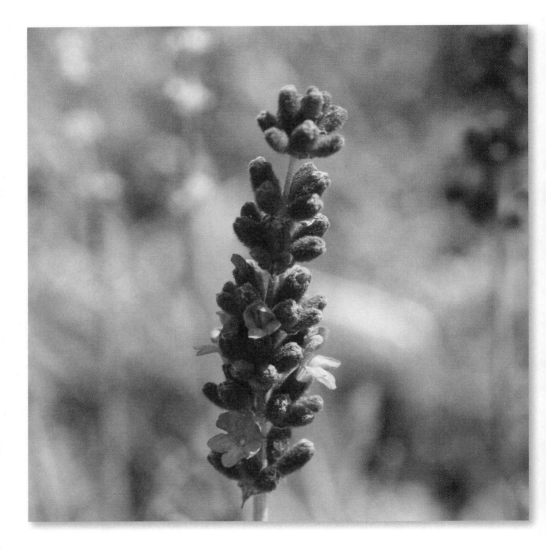

Introduction

Go to your fields and your gardens, and you shall learn
that it is the pleasure of the bee to gather honey of the
flower,
But it is also the pleasure of the flower to yield its honey to
the bee.
For to the bee a flower is a fountain of life,
And to the flower a bee is a messenger of love,
And to both, bee and flower, the giving and the receiving of
pleasure is a need and an ecstasy.

KAHLIL GIBRAN, "ON PLEASURE"

This book provides a comprehensive overview of the protective, restorative, "scentual" qualities and properties of essential oils and their role as guardians of wellness and well-being. It is aimed at those who are interested in using essential oils in their everyday lives, and it also serves as a useful reference guide for students, health-care professionals, and any therapists who wish to apply essential oils safely within their practice. Much of the information is presented in the form of tables, charts, and diagrams for ease of reading and usage.

We'll begin with an overview of the body's anatomy and functional systems so that the reader may understand how the body absorbs and eliminates essential oils, how they may provoke an emotional and/or physiological response, and how to appropriately apply them. Then we'll move on to safety concerns, a protocol for creating effective essential oil blends, and the multidynamic qualities and characteristics of essential oils, including their subtle elements and energies.

Some information inevitably crosses over from my first book, *Essential Oils for Mindfulness and Meditation,* particularly in relation to safe practice. This book, *Essential Oils for the Whole Body,* exponentially "grows" the reader's knowledge and understanding of essential oils. You'll find here more detail, deeper insight, and broader guidance for the application and healing potential of aromatherapy. My hope is that this book can be your go-to handbook for the appropriate and effective application of essential oils in healing therapies.

The Serenity Essential Oils

Of the 400 aromatic species used as essential oils, I have designated fifteen as Serenity Essential Oils. They are among the least hazardous and most helpful essential oils, and they complement and support one another's properties well, from encouraging a sense of calm, focus, and concentration during meditation and relaxation techniques to invaluable antimicrobial, skin-soothing, and rejuvenating properties. Indeed, as a group, these fifteen essential oils serve as a well-rounded, comprehensive, and powerful tool kit for healing and aromatherapy.

The Serenity Essential Oils are:

Cajeput *(Melaleuca cajuputi)*

Carrot seed *(Daucus carota)*

Chamomile, German and Roman *(Matricaria recutita, Anthemis nobilis)*

Cypress *(Cupressus sempervirens)*

Frankincense *(Boswellia carterii, B. sacra)*

Galbanum *(Ferula galbaniflua)*

Geranium *(Pelargonium graveolens, P. × asperum)*

Lavender, English and spike *(Lavandula angustifolia, L. latifolia)*

Mandarin *(Citrus reticulata)*

Patchouli *(Pogostemon cablin)*

Petitgrain *(Citrus aurantium* var. *amara)*

Rose otto *(Rosa* × *centifolia, R.* × *damascena)*

Spikenard *(Nardostachys jatamansi, N. grandiflora)*

Tea tree *(Melaleuca alternifolia)*

Vetivert *(Vetiveria zizanioides)*

There are three types of mandarin (red, yellow, and green). While their qualities are all very similar, my personal preference is for green; I find its perfume notes and qualities lend themselves well to the other Serenity Essential Oils. Therefore, you will notice that I refer to green mandarin in the lists and charts. You can, of course, use the other types of mandarin if you prefer.

Pure rose otto essential oil is very expensive to produce. It is, however, available for purchase as a 5% blend diluted in jojoba oil. While my preference is to use pure essential oils, I do, in the case of rose, include information about rose absolute too. As you will discover, absolutes contain residues of the solvent used to extract essential oil from the plant material (in this case, petals), and are thus prone to cause sensitization. For this reason, my preference is definitely to use pure rose otto essential oil for skin care preparations (in massage oils, creams, and lotions, for example). However, rose absolute exudes beautiful notes that work equally well psycho-emotionally, when diffused and when making aesthetic perfumes, and aids affordability too, as it's less expensive to purchase. In either case, rose is very highly perfumed, so can be used in extreme moderation.

1

Anatomy

Building Blocks of the Human Body

This chapter provides a brief foundational description of the body and its various systems, starting, of course, with the cell, the basic building block of the human body. Knowing how the body develops and functions as an interactive unit, you will have a better understanding of how essential oils behave and how their molecules are absorbed and interact within the body.

Cells are the smallest unit of life, but atoms are the smallest unit of matter. Matter (which is defined as physical substance) consists of various types of particles, the most familiar being the electron, the proton, and the neuron. These subatomic particles variously combine to form atoms. Atoms with the same kind of constituent arrangement of particles group together to form unique elements: there are more than a hundred different kinds of atoms, creating more than a hundred different unique chemical elements. A combination of atoms forms molecules. Atoms and/or molecules can come together to create a compound. Cells consist of an array of large molecules. But how does this relate to the formation of the human body? Let's take a closer look.

Building the Human Body

ATOMS
- The basic building block of everything.
- The smallest unit of matter that participates in chemical reactions; cannot

be naturally broken down without release of an electrically charged particle; cannot be subdivided without destroying its identity.

- Arranged as a central nucleus surrounded by electrons.
- Central nucleus is made up of two particles: protons and neutrons.
- Electrons have a negative charge. Protons have a positive charge. Neutrons carry no charge. In an atom with an equal number of electrons and protons, the negative and positive charges cancel each other out.
- Electrons, protons, and neutrons are known as subatomic particles.
- The mass number of an atom is the total number of neutrons and protons it contains.
- The nucleus of an atom is extremely small; atoms comprise mainly empty space.
- Atoms measure approximately one hundred millionth of a centimeter in diameter.

ELEMENTS

- The simplest substances.
- Cannot be broken down into a simpler form capable of independent existence as observable matter.
- Made up completely of atoms of only one kind.
- Basic substances from which all others derive, built up by chemical combination.
- Ninety-two elements occur naturally (twenty less stable elements have been created through nuclear physics); all elements are set out and represented on the periodic table.
- The elements carbon, hydrogen, oxygen, and nitrogen make up 96 percent of all living things.

MOLECULES

- Simplest unit of a chemical compound that can exist in a free state, consisting of two or more atoms held together by chemical bonds.
- Two types: *homonuclear molecules* consist of atoms of a singular chemical element—e.g., molecular oxygen (O_2, or two oxygen atoms joined together); *heteronuclear molecules* consist of more than one

element—e.g., water (H_2O, or two hydrogen atoms joined with an oxygen atom).

COMPOUNDS

- Chemical substances whose molecules are made up of two or more different elements that have become chemically bonded or joined together. For example:

    Water (H_2O) is a compound of the elements hydrogen and oxygen.

    Carbon dioxide (CO_2) is a compound of the elements carbon and oxygen.

    Table salt (NaCl) is a compound of the elements sodium and chlorine.

- When elements are joined to form a compound, the atoms that comprise them lose their individual properties and the compound takes on its own unique and defined chemical structure.

THE MAIN CHEMICAL ELEMENTS FOUND WITHIN THE BODY

ELEMENT (CHEMICAL SYMBOL)	PERCENTAGE OF TOTAL BODY MASS
Oxygen (O)	65.0
Carbon (C)	18.5
Hydrogen (H)	9.5
Nitrogen (N)	3.2
Calcium (Ca)	1.5
Phosphorus (P)	1.0
Potassium (K)	0.35
Sulfur (S)	0.25
Sodium (Na)	0.2
Chlorine (Cl)	0.2
Magnesium (Mg)	0.1
Iron (Fe)	0.005

TRACE ELEMENTS (CHEMICAL SYMBOL)	PERCENTAGE OF TOTAL BODY MASS
Aluminium (Al), boron (B), chromium (Cr), cobalt (Co), copper (Cu), fluorine (F), iodine (I), manganese (Mn), molybdenum (Mo), selenium (Se), silicon (Si), tin (Sn), vanadium (V), zinc (Zn)	0.195–0.2

CELLS

Molecules combine to form cells, which are the smallest functional units of the body (they are too small to be seen with the naked eye). Humans are made up of eukaryotic cells, meaning that our cells contain a nucleus and organelles. (Prokaryotic cells, in contrast, do not contain a nucleus and organelles. These types of cells are typical of bacteria.) The mitochondria organelles within a eukaryotic cell convert nutrients into energy. Specialized types of cells perform specific functions and relay information to one another.

+ **Exocrine cells** secrete fluids such as sweat and enzymes.
+ **Epithelial cells** on the skin's surface and within the body provide protection and absorb nutrients.
+ **Endocrine cells** secrete hormones into the bloodstream.
+ **Blood cells** deliver oxygen throughout the body; they also aid in the elimination of waste and fight infection.

Cellular metabolism, sometimes called cellular respiration, is the process by which cells consume and release energy. During the process of cellular respiration, molecules (nutrients) are broken down into smaller units to release and convert biochemical energy into adenosine triphosphate (ATP). Glucose is the main nutrient to fuel this process. Carbohydrates, amino acids, and fatty acid molecules are also used but to a lesser extent. Energy released as a result of this process is used to power cellular activity, and some is stored.

Oxygen potentiates cellular respiration by helping to create and transport energy in its molecules. Water helps as well; cells are 65 to

90 percent water, and drinking sufficient water can help keep them functioning at optimal levels.

The Structure of the Cell

A cell consists of a plasma membrane, inside which are a number of organelles floating in a watery fluid called cytosol. The inner aspect, contained within the plasma membrane but not part of the nucleus, is known as the cytoplasm.

Organelles are structures within a cell that perform highly specialized functions. They include the following:

- **Nucleus**—storehouse of the organism's genetic material in the form of DNA.
- **Mitochondria**—the energy powerhouse of the cell; they produce ATP and regulate cell metabolism.
- **Ribosomes**—facilitate protein synthesis.
- **Endoplasmic reticulum**—facilitates the transport of materials within the cell.

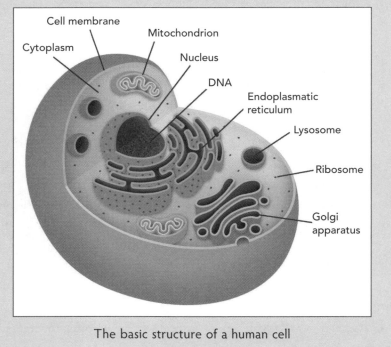

The basic structure of a human cell

> • **Golgi apparatus**—facilitates the modification and transport of proteins within the cell.
> • **Lysosomes**—contain digestive enzymes to break down waste, including dead cells.

Integrity of the organism is maintained partly by cell division; as cells die, they are continuously replaced with new ones. This process occurs in two ways: mitosis and meiosis.

✦ **Mitosis:** Each chromosome in a cell nucleus divides into two. The nucleus then divides to contain each set of chromosomes, and this is followed by division of cytoplasm, organelles, and then cell membrane to produce two identical cells. Through mitosis, the body produces new cells for growth, repair, and the replacement of older cells. Some cells are replaced rapidly (over thirty to ninety minutes, in some instances); for example, hair, skin, fingernails, taste buds, and the lining of the stomach are replaced constantly at a rapid rate throughout life. On the other hand, brain cells and nerve cells in the central nervous system are often reproduced only in the first few months of life.

✦ **Meiosis:** When division occurs in reproductive cells, the number of chromosomes is reduced to half in each new cell: the ovum (female egg cell) and the spermatozoon (male sperm cell). The union of an ovum and spermatozoon (fertilization) creates a single cell, called the zygote. The zygote rapidly divides (mitosis) and multiplies, and each new cell created through this process possesses the same genetic makeup as the originating zygote cell. In this way a new organism is created containing equal amounts of genetic material from the ovum and the spermatozoon.

BODY TISSUES

Cells in the body come together to form tissues with specific functions. There are four basic types:

+ **Epithelial tissue,** a membrane-like tissue, covers free surfaces and lines cavities and tubes in the body.
+ **Connective tissue** can be semisolid and jelly-like or dense and rigid, depending on the function of the tissue. As its name implies, connective tissue serves to connect (enlace, support, or sheathe) other tissues. It is found in all organs of the body and within blood.
+ **Muscle tissue** is contractile, meaning it can shorten and allow movement.
+ **Nervous tissue,** the main tissue of the nervous system, conveys electrical impulses to and from the brain and throughout the body.

ORGANS

Different tissues are grouped together to form organs, which have specific functions and usually recognizable shapes—consider, for example, the stomach, heart, liver, lungs, and brain. Organs are grouped together to form physiological systems with specific functions. For example, the digestive system comprises tubing that originates at the mouth and ends at the anus, with connection to supporting organs such as the gallbladder, liver, and pancreas, and is responsible for breaking down and absorbing nutrients from food.

Cell
(the smallest functional unit)
⬇
Tissue
(epithelial, connective, muscle, nervous)
⬇
Organs
(brain, heart, lungs, liver, gallbladder, kidneys, stomach, pancreas, spleen, duodenum, large and small intestines, colon, uterus, ovaries/testes)
⬇

Organ systems
(integumentary, skeletal, muscular, nervous,
endocrine, cardiovascular, lymphatic,
immune, respiratory, digestive, urinary,
excretory, reproductive)

THE ORGAN SYSTEMS OF THE BODY

Integumentary System

Components/Organs

The integumentary system is the skin and the structures derived from it, such as hair, nails, sweat glands, and oil glands. It is composed mainly of two layers: the epidermis and dermis.

The epidermis is the superficial layer of the skin. It contains melanocytes that contribute to the absorption of UV light and the color of the skin (and also the hair and iris of the eye). It also contains keratinocytes; these cells produce keratin, a fibrous protein that strengthens the skin, hair, and nails. The epidermis can itself be broken down into its component layers:

+ **Stratum corneum:** Twenty-five to thirty layers of dead skin cells, which are constantly being shed. (These superficial layers of skin help prevent the penetration of microbes and dehydration of underlying tissues.)
+ **Stratum lucidum:** Three to five layers of flattened keratinocytes; present only in the skin of the fingertips, palms, and soles of the feet.
+ **Stratum granulosum:** Three to five layers of flattened keratinocytes in which organelles are beginning to degenerate.
+ **Stratum spinosum:** Eight to ten rows of many-sided healthy keratinocytes, formed as a result of cell division in the stratum basale.
+ **Stratum basale** (also called **stratum germinativum**): This basal or deepest layer is composed of a single row of cuboidal or columnar keratinocytes. New skin cells are made in this layer.

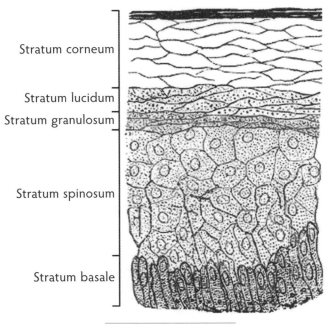

Stratum corneum

Stratum lucidum
Stratum granulosum

Stratum spinosum

Stratum basale

Layers of the epidermis

The dermis, or "true skin," contains adipose tissue (fat), blood vessels, lymph vessels, nerve endings, sweat glands, and hair follicles (see diagram on page 51). It is thickest on the heels of the palms and the soles of the feet, and thinnest on the eyelids and skull. Comprised of collagen fibers, the dermis is tough and elastic; however, it can rupture when overstretched, leaving permanent stretch marks (for example, in pregnancy, obesity, or muscle building).

Function
+ Protects the body and internal organs.
+ Acts as a barrier against pathogens (bacteria and viruses).
+ Offers some protection against UV light.
+ Offers limited absorption properties—e.g., some fat-soluble substances (like oxygen, carbon dioxide, steroid hormones, and vitamins A, D, E, and K), resins and some essential oils, organic solvents (e.g., paint thinner), and salts of heavy metals (such as lead, mercury, or nickel).

✦ Assists in the formation of vitamin D.

✦ Assists the regulation of body temperature.

✦ Eliminates metabolic wastes (via sweat).

✦ Detects and relays sensory information, such as touch, pressure, pain, warmth, and cold.

Skeletal System
Components/Organs
The skeletal system includes not just the 206 bones of the human body but also its cartilage and ligaments. Bones are about 20 percent water, 30 to 40 percent organic material, and 40 to 50 percent inorganic material (mineral salts, mainly calcium and phosphorus).

Function

✦ Supports and maintains the body's structure (framework).

✦ Protects vital organs.

✦ Aids body movements by giving leverage to muscle attachments.

✦ Produces red and white blood cells within red marrow; stores fat in yellow marrow.

✦ Stores minerals (calcium phosphate, calcium carbonate, phosphorus, magnesium, sodium) in bone tissues.

Muscular System
Components/Organs
Muscle cells are organized and develop into different types of muscular tissue (some microscopic), as follows:

✦ Myofilaments (formed from the proteins actin and myosin)

✦ Myofibrils (muscle fibers)

✦ Fasciculi (muscle bundles)

✦ Muscles and muscle groups (e.g., the biceps in the upper arm, and the rhomboids major and minor in the upper back)

Muscle fibers form different types of muscle structures depending on their location and function:

+ **Smooth muscles** form the walls of hollow organs (e.g., the stomach, bladder, and blood vessels) and facilitate the transportation of materials, moving them along or restricting their flow.
+ **Cardiac muscles** are an involuntary, striated muscle fibers that forms the walls of the heart.
+ **Skeletal muscles** are attached to bones or related structures and stimulated by nerve impulses to move the skeleton.

Function

+ Allows external mobility—that is, moving the body, whether lifting a finger, shifting in your seat, or running.
+ Allows internal mobility—that is, movement resulting from contraction of smooth muscle, like peristalsis of the intestines.
+ Controls posture, stabilizing the body.
+ Generates heat through muscle contraction and movement—when the body becomes cold, muscles contract rapidly (shivering) to produce heat to maintain a suitable core temperature.

Nervous System

Components/Organs

The nervous system is one of the two specialized control centers (the other being the endocrine system) that mediate body processes in order to maintain homeostasis. It is the master control and communication system and consists of two main parts: the central nervous system and peripheral nervous system.

+ **The central nervous system (CNS),** comprising the brain and spinal cord, is concerned with interpreting incoming sensory information and issuing instructions in the form of motor responses, as well as being the control center for thoughts and emotions.
+ **The peripheral nervous system (PNS)** comprises all the nerves that branch off from the brain and spinal cord and extend throughout the rest of the body. There are forty-three pairs of PNS nerves: twelve pairs of cranial nerves and thirty-one pairs of spinal nerves. The PNS is divided into two distinct functional

aspects: the **somatic nervous system** (which controls voluntary movement of skeletal muscles) and the **autonomic nervous system** (which controls involuntary impulses to smooth muscle tissue).

The autonomic nervous system is further divided into the **sympathetic nervous system** and the **parasympathetic nervous system,** which operate complementarily with each other. The sympathetic system stimulates, while the parasympathetic system calms or reduces. For example, when we are faced with a threat, fear stimulates the sympathetic nervous system to release hormones that increase the heart rate and focus mental alertness. Then, once the perceived threat is no longer prominent, the parasympathetic nervous system releases hormones that counterbalance this reaction, slowing the heart rate to restore a normal functional state of physiological calmness and equilibrium.

Function

+ Provides sensory input: sensory receptors, like olfactory receptor neurons, detect and respond to stimuli (internal or external) such as pressure, temperature, and motion.
+ Interprets and responds to stimuli: the nervous system interprets sensory information and responds by sending nerve impulses, causing muscular contractions or glandular secretions.
+ Controls higher mental functioning and emotional responsiveness: the nervous system is responsible for mental processes, such as cognition and memory, and emotional responses, such as joy, anger, frustration, anxiety, excitement, and fear.

Essential oils, especially when applied in conjunction with appropriate touch through massage (including self-massage), regulate and calm the nervous system by provoking positive parasympathetic nervous system responses.

Endocrine System

Components/Organs

The second major control and communication system of the body, the endocrine system governs the glands of the body that produce hormones to regulate such processes as growth, development, metabolism, sleep, and mood. Its structures include:

+ The glands—pituitary, pineal, thyroid, parathyroid, thymus, adrenals, pancreas, and gonads
+ The products of the glands—that is, hormones
+ The feedback loops by which the body modulates hormone release to maintain homeostasis

Function

+ Produces and secretes hormones.
+ Regulates physiological activities such as growth, development, and metabolism.
+ Helps the body adapt during times of stress—for example, through release of glucocorticoids, including cortisol, from the adrenals to help mediate the stress response)—e.g., during infection, trauma, dehydration, emotional stress, or starvation.
+ Contributes to the process of reproduction.

Cardiovascular, Lymphatic, and Immune Systems

The body is mostly fluid, which varies in its composition depending on its location and function within the body. For example:

+ **Extracellular fluid** is situated between the cells.
+ **Interstitial fluid** is located between tissues.
+ **Plasma** is located within the blood.
+ **Lymph** circulates through the lymphatic system.

The cardiovascular, lymphatic, and immune systems all have their basis in the body's fluids. The cardiovascular system pumps blood around the body to circulate oxygen, nutrients, and hormones to tissues and organs. The lymphatic system is a one-way drainage system designed to remove excess fluid from the body's tissues, and it works complementarily with the cardiovascular system. Both systems support immunity.

The cardiovascular system comprises:

+ **Blood:** This liquid connective tissue brings nutrients and oxygen to body tissues. It consists of plasma, platelets, and white and red blood cells.

+ **Blood vessels:** Arteries carry blood away from the heart, while veins carry blood back to the heart. Threadlike capillaries have thin, semipermeable walls and spread throughout the body's tissues. They provide oxygen and nutrients to the surrounding tissue and remove cellular waste from interstitial fluid.

+ **Heart:** The heart contains four hollow chambers (two atria, two ventricles) that function as a double pump: the right-hand pump forces deoxygenated blood to the lungs (for gaseous exchange, releasing carbon dioxide and absorbing oxygen), while the left-hand pump forces oxygen-rich blood to the rest of the body.

The lymphatic system is a circulatory system that removes fluids and proteins that have escaped from cells and tissues and returns them to the blood, in the process filtering out waste. It comprises:

+ **Lymph:** the fluid carried by the lymph system
+ **Lymphatic vessels:** the vessels that transport lymph throughout the body
+ **Lymphoid tissues:** glands and nodes that filter lymph; they tend to be clustered in the neck, armpits, abdomen, groin, and elbow and knee joints
+ **Lymphoid organs:** the tonsils, adenoids, spleen, and thymus, which filter lymph and produce immune cells—T cells from the thymus, for example, and lymphocytes from the spleen

Transportation of lymph depends entirely on pressure to the vessel walls, which is initiated by physical pressure, the milking action of skeletal muscle contraction, or changes in pressure in the thorax and abdomen during breathing. In other words, exercise, massage, and deep breathing stimulate the lymphatic system.

Function of the Cardiovascular System
+ Transports respiratory gases (e.g., oxygen, carbon dioxide).
+ Transports nutrients from the digestive tract.

+ Transports antibodies, waste materials, and hormones from endocrine glands.
+ Transports heat from active muscles to the skin, where it dissipates (via perspiration, vasodilation), facilitating temperature regulation.
+ Supports immune function by circulating white blood cells.
+ Supports immune function by transporting pathogens and impurities to filtration sites.
+ Prevents hemorrhage and loss of body fluids through blood clotting (platelets clumping together).

Function of the Lymphatic System

+ Drains excess interstitial fluid from the tissues, returning it to the cardiovascular system, thereby maintaining blood volume and pressure and preventing swelling (edema).
+ Transports fatty acids, fats (chyle), and some vitamins from the digestive tract to the blood.
+ Returns proteins and cellular debris that have escaped from the blood back into general circulation.
+ Transports white blood cells to and from the lymph nodes; transports antigen-presenting cells (APCs), such as dendritic cells, to the lymph nodes, where an immune response is stimulated.
+ Supports the immune response through filtration and destruction of disease organisms via lymphocytes and antibodies.

Respiratory System

Components/Organs

Together with the cardiovascular system, the respiratory system ensures the constant supply of oxygen to body tissues and the elimination of carbon dioxide. Without oxygen, cells die (within five minutes). With too much carbon dioxide in the blood, the body's pH becomes acidic, beginning a chain of bad reactions. For these reasons, respiration is vital to homeostasis. The system consists of the following:

+ **Nasal cavity:** Hollow space inside the nose and skull terminating in the throat. It is lined with hairs and a mucous membrane and its function is to condition air—that is, to warm, moisten, and filter it—before it reaches the lungs.

✦ **Pharynx (throat):** Muscular tubing (shared with the digestive tract) extending from behind the nasal cavity to the back of the oral cavity and down to the laryngopharynx. It contains the tonsils, lymphatic organs that support the immune system by protecting against inhaled or ingested pathogens.

✦ **Larynx (voice box):** The upper part of the trachea formed by cartilage and containing the vocal cords (bands of elastic ligaments attached by skeletal muscle to the rigid cartilage of the larynx).

✦ **Trachea (windpipe):** A membraneceous tube supported by rings of cartilage extending from the larynx to the upper chest, where it divides into the right and left bronchi. It conveys air into and out of the lungs.

✦ **Bronchi:** Large, tube-like air-conducting passageways, reinforced with cartilage, leading from the trachea to each lung, where they branch out like tree roots, forming smaller bronchioles.

✦ **Alveoli:** Tiny, very thin sacs, comprising a blend of epithelial and elastic connective tissue, attached to the ends of the bronchioles and surrounded by a network of capillaries. Here gaseous exchange takes place: carbon dioxide leaves the blood, passing from the capillaries to the alveoli, and oxygen enters it, passing from the alveoli to the capillaries. There are approximately 300 million alveoli, which provide a collective surface area of around 1,000 square feet.

✦ **Lungs:** The highly elastic and spongy organs of respiration. The right lung has three lobes, and the left lung two (to accommodate space in the chest for the heart). Serous membranes line the external surface of each lung, and both are encased by the pleural membrane, which secretes a thin serous fluid that minimizes friction and allows easy movement of the lungs during respiration.

✦ **Respiratory diaphragm:** The main muscle of respiration, a dome-shaped muscular band that is attached to the lower ribs and spine and separates the thoracic cavity from the abdominal cavity.

Function

+ Permits respiration and gaseous exchange of carbon dioxide and oxygen.
+ Allows vocal sounds: air exhaled from the lungs flows through the vocal cords, which, when consciously controlled, produces sound.
+ Enables the sense of smell: air drawn up through the nose comes into contact with the olfactory epithelium, initiating the olfactory process (see chapter 2).

Digestive System

Components/Organs

Digestion is the process by which food molecules are broken down (refined) into usable units in preparation for assimilation by the body. Usable nutrients are delivered to vital organs via the circulatory system; unusable waste products are excreted as feces. The digestive system follows the path of the alimentary canal, or gastrointestinal tract, a long hollow tube that begins at the mouth and ends at the anus. It includes the following:

+ Mouth
+ Esophagus
+ Stomach
+ Small intestine (divided into the duodenum, jejunum, and ileum)
+ Large intestine (a.k.a. the colon)
+ Rectum
+ Anus

The liver, gallbladder, and pancreas play important roles in the digestive system. Among other things, they do the following:

+ **Liver:** Processes nutrients from food; produces bile, which breaks down fats in foods; stores energy from food in the form of glycogen.
+ **Gallbladder:** Stores bile produced by the liver and secretes it into the small intestine as needed.
+ **Pancreas:** Secretes enzymes that break down food into the small intestine; secretes insulin into the bloodstream, which helps the body regulate blood sugar levels as it metabolizes food.

Function

+ Converts food into nutrients and energy for the body.
+ Allows the absorption and assimilation of nutrients from food.
+ Filters and eliminates indigestible materials and waste products of digestion and other body processes.

Urinary/Excretory System

Components/Organs

The excretory system integrates the urinary system with all the other excretory organs of the body. The urinary system includes the following:

+ Kidneys
+ Ureter and urethra
+ Bladder

But urine is not the only vehicle by which waste leaves the body. Other components of the body's excretory system include the following:

+ Integumentary system (sweat from the skin)
+ Digestive system (feces)
+ Respiratory system (heat and carbon dioxide)
+ Eyes (tears), nose (mucus), ears (earwax)

The bean-shaped kidneys, situated to the left and right in the upper lumbar region of the spine, filter metabolic waste, excess ions, and chemicals from the blood as it passes through. They dump these wastes into the urine and feed it to the ureters, ducts that convey urine to the bladder for storage and then excretion through the urethra.

Function

+ Filters metabolic waste from blood and excretes it in urine (and sweat, mucus, tears, et cetera).
+ Regulates blood pH by monitoring and controlling levels of hydrogen and bicarbonate ions in the blood, filtering them out and allowing reabsorption as needed.
+ Continually monitors and manages blood pressure, secreting or releasing enzymes to stimulate vasoconstriction (contraction of

the muscle wall of blood vessels) and controlling the balance of fluid through retention or excretion to manage blood volume.

Reproductive System

Components/Organs

The reproductive system consists of the following:

+ Gonads (ovaries in females, testes in males)
+ Ducts (fallopian tubes in females, spermatic ducts in males)
+ Gametes (ova in females, spermatozoa in males)
+ Reproductive organs (uterus and vagina in females, penis and prostate gland in males)

Gonads are reproductive glands, located in the pelvic cavity in women and scrotum in males, that produce gametes (specialized sex cells) capable of fusing together to form a new organism (that is, fusion of the female ovum and the male spermatozoon to form an embryo). Gonads also release hormones that stimulate and regulate reproductive and other bodily processes, such as the growth and development of primary sex organs (genitalia) and secondary sex characteristics. For example:

+ In males, the testes release testosterone, which produces an increase in body hair (especially facial, underarm, abdominal, chest, and pubic) and increased size and mass of muscles, bones, and vocal cords.
+ In females, the ovaries release estrogen, which stimulates the development of breasts and widening of the hips, increases body fat distribution (especially in the hips, thighs, buttocks, and breasts), and initiates the process of menstruation.

Function

+ Propagates the species by producing offspring.
+ Defines male and female physiology and characteristics.
+ Releases pheromones to stimulate sexual attraction to enhance the possibility of reproduction.

2

Absorption

Pathways into the Body

This chapter explores the three routes by which the body absorbs essential oils:

✦ Olfaction (inhalation)
✦ Percutaneous (skin) absorption
✦ Oral ingestion

It also discusses the influence of specific essential oils on our psychological, emotional, and physiological state.

OLFACTION (INHALATION)

The term *olfaction* refers to our sense of smell. You might argue that smelling essential oils—that is, inhalation—is actually a form of ingestion, but I tend to think of it as a topical application. Like topical applications to the skin, olfaction allows only limited absorption of essential oils into the body (unlike oral ingestion, which allows 100 percent absorption). However, unlike skin applications, olfaction serves as a gateway to the lungs and brain, and when we inhale essential oils, they can stimulate very powerful effects on our body and psyche. Furthermore, given the highly volatile, odiferous nature of essential oils, all methods of topical application also trigger our sense of smell and thus, by default, involve olfaction as a delivery route.

The Sense of Smell

Chemical molecules exuding from an essential oil (or from essential oils released from oil glands in plants) readily combine with oxygen molecules in the surrounding atmosphere as they evaporate. When we inhale, we draw in that oxygen-rich air that is impregnated with essential oil molecules; it flows up our nasal cavities and sweeps across the olfactory epithelium before being redirected down the trachea (windpipe) and into the lungs.

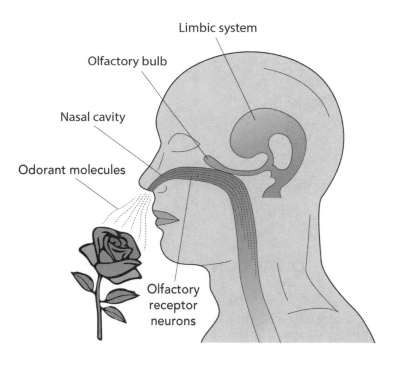

The olfactory system

The olfactory epithelium occupies about 2.5 to 3 square centimeters at the top of the nasal cavity. It contains three types of cells: olfactory receptor neurons, basal cells (which continuously generate new receptor neurons), and supporting cells. The epithelium is covered by a lipid-rich, yellow-tinted mucous membrane that measures about 60 microns thick, constantly flows, and is replaced approximately every ten minutes. The mucous membrane contains enzymes, mucopolysaccharides, salts, and antibodies that prevent infectious microorganisms from passing into the brain via the porous ethmoid bone, which separates the brain from the nasal cavity.

At one end of each olfactory receptor neuron, hairlike cilia extend into the mucous membrane that covers the epithelium. The cilia are covered with receptors, which function like a lock-and-key mechanism; when the right key (an odorant molecule) is matched to the lock (the receptor), the mechanism is activated. At the other end of the neuron, an axon (nerve fiber) extends upward, quickly joining with axons from other receptor cells to form branches of the olfactory nerve. These branches pass through the porous ethmoid bone and terminate in the olfactory bulb, the bulbous anterior projection of the olfactory lobe in the forebrain.

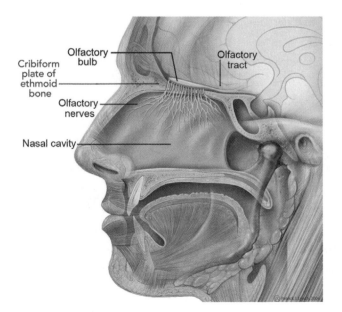

Odorant molecules carried within the air we inhale are captured by the mucous lining, which acts as a solvent to break them down. There, depending on their molecular shape, they "lock" with specific receptors on the cilia, thereby activating them. Upon receiving notice that their cilia receptors have been activated, the olfactory receptor neurons convert (transduce) that activation into electrical impulses that are relayed along the olfactory nerves to mitral cells in the left and right olfactory bulbs. The mitral cells relay those neural impulses deeper into the brain via nerve bundles known as the olfactory tracts. Those tracts converge at the anterior commissure, a band of nerve tissue that is situated beneath the frontal lobe in front of the columns of the fornix, and connects the left and right hemispheres of the brain. Along the way, the neural signals are sent to target receptive areas within the brain that collectively form the limbic system.

The Three Evolutionary States of Brain Development

The brain is perhaps easiest to understand when we put it within the context of its evolution. According to the triune brain theory of evolution, the human brain developed in three stages:

- **The primitive or "reptilian" brain,** which includes the brainstem and its structures, controls our most basic physiology: the autonomic nervous system, which controls our heart rate, digestion, respiration, and other vital processes, as well as our instinctual responses to stress, sex, reproduction, and so on—including sensory stimulation like olfaction.
- **The intermediate or "paleomammalian" brain,** meaning the limbic system, controls our psycho-emotional response to our environment.
- **The superior or "neomammalian" brain** came about with the development of the neocortex, including the prefrontal cortex, which facilitates mental and intellectual functions such as language, abstract thought, reasoning, imagination, short- and long-term memory, and so on.

These three brains are distinct yet integrated in function. As you'll see in the pages that follow, olfaction, as a system for interpreting sensory input, which was a vital process for the reptilian brain and contributed to our most basic survival instincts, evolved in step with the human brain, becoming one of our most valuable tools for engaging with the world and ourselves.

The Limbic System

The "limbic system" is not actually a separate *system* but the collective label given to a complex group of structures found within the center of the brain, lying on either side of the thalamus, that closely interface with each other and work as a functional unit, supporting the processes involved with emotions, behavior, and motivation. Four of its components form two C-shaped structures in the brain—one made up of the hippocampus and the fornix, the other made up of the cingulate gyrus and the parahippocampal gyrus. It also includes the hypothalamus, mammillary body, and amygdala.

The limbic system operates by influencing and stimulating the autonomic nervous system (part of the primitive reptilian brain) and the endocrine system. It is directly connected to the prefrontal cortex (part of the neomammalian brain) via signals relayed by dopaminergic neurotransmitters from the thalamus. Dopamine is a chemical released by nerve cells to send signals to other nerve cells in the brain and other parts of the body. The prefrontal cortex is where the brain makes sense of, identifies, rationalizes, reasons, categorizes, and decides in relation

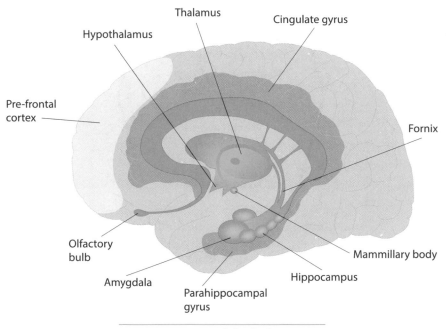

Major structures of the limbic system

to emotional and instinctual messages received from the limbic system (and other sensory systems such as sight, hearing, and touch).

Because the limbic system is so greatly influenced by the olfaction pathway, it plays an important role in the dynamics of therapeutic applications of essential oils. Let's look at some of its structures and functions.

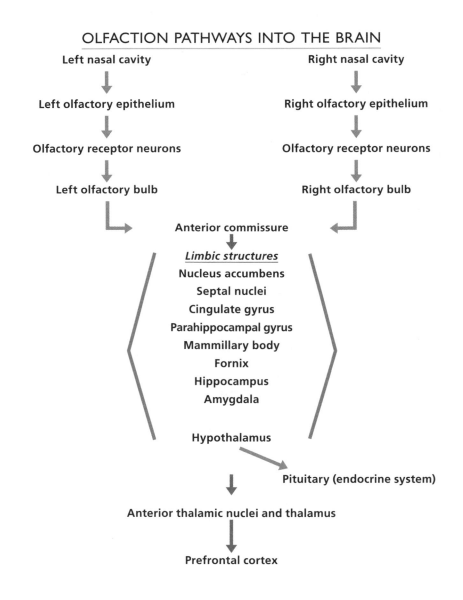

OLFACTION PATHWAYS INTO THE BRAIN

Left nasal cavity · Right nasal cavity

Left olfactory epithelium · Right olfactory epithelium

Olfactory receptor neurons · Olfactory receptor neurons

Left olfactory bulb · Right olfactory bulb

Anterior commissure

Limbic structures
Nucleus accumbens
Septal nuclei
Cingulate gyrus
Parahippocampal gyrus
Mammillary body
Fornix
Hippocampus
Amygdala

Hypothalamus

Pituitary (endocrine system)

Anterior thalamic nuclei and thalamus

Prefrontal cortex

Olfactory Tubercle

The olfactory tubercle, part of the olfactory structures in the basal forebrain, receives signals from the olfactory bulb and is interconnected with sensory arousal and reward centers within the brain. It is thought to function as a significant interface between processing sensory information and subsequent behavioral responses (especially those relating to attentional behaviors and social and sensory responsiveness).

Thalamus

The thalamus is a dense mass of nerve cells roughly similar in size and shape to a walnut. The two halves of the thalamus "walnut" sit on either side of the lateral wall of the third ventricle, in close proximity to each other. The thalamus receives input from the sensory organs, including the skin, as well as the internal organs, especially the intestines. It relays neural signals to the frontal lobe and other areas within the cerebral cortex.

In the brain, nuclei are clusters of nerve cells with specific functions. The anterior thalamic nuclei are a base of connectivity for the limbic system and the prefrontal cortex. They are thought to play a role in the modulation of alertness, learning, and episodic memory and may also contribute to reciprocal hippocampal-prefrontal interactions involved in emotional and executive functions.

Hypothalamus

The hypothalamus is situated at the front edge of and just below the thalamus. It is approximately the size of a pea and is linked to the nervous and endocrine system via the pituitary gland. The hypothalamus is concerned with the internal environment of the body and basic instinctive undifferentiated emotions (anger, sorrow, pleasure, displeasure). The hypothalamus controls hunger, thirst, body temperature, circadian rhythms, and aspects of attachment and parenting behaviors. It regulates the functioning of the autonomic nervous system and is involved in memory, including scent memory and recognition, as well as the motivational and emotional aspects of smell.

Amygdala

The amygdala is either of two almond-shaped bundles of nuclei situated almost centrally in each brain hemisphere, in close proximity to each other. They receive signals from all the sensory systems, including the olfactory bulb and other olfactory structures, and are involved in the sense of smell and pheromone procesing. They are tightly connected to the hypothalamus by numerous nerve bundles, and they act to control hypothalamic drives and provide an emotional window into the external environment on behalf of the hypothalamus. The hypothalamus is concerned with autonomic instinct, but the amygdalae selectively discriminate and are involved with memory and the modulation of memory consolidation, decision making, and emotional reactions. Impairment of the amygdalae (which can be caused by overexposure to stress, among other things) can lead to prolonged and "learned" negative states of aggression, fear, and anxiety and may lead to conditions such as post-traumatic stress disorder (PTSD) and obsessive compulsive disorder (OCD). Meditation—especially mindfulness meditation—has been shown to modulate the amygdalae and may lead to and support feelings of acceptance and social connectedness.

Hippocampus

The human brain has two hippocampi, one on each side. Each is a curving elongated ridge that extends over the floor of the descending horn of each lateral ventricle of the brain. The hippocampus is concerned with processing events and experiences into memory (including scent memory). The hippocampus also contains "place cells" that help us recognize and orient our location within the external environment. Damage to or deterioration of the hippocampus is associated with the memory impairment that occurs with Alzheimer's disease.

Fornix

The fornix is a C-shaped bundle of fibers that carry signals from the hippocampus to the hypothalamus; *posterior* fibers continue to the mammillary bodies and then to the anterior nuclei of the thalamus, while *anterior* fibers continue to the septal nuclei and nucleus accumbens.

Mammillary Body

A mammillary body is either of two small, round bodies that project from the posterior hypothalamus. They act as relays for impulses from the amygdalae and hippocampi to the anterior nuclei of the thalamus. Mammillary bodies are involved with our recognition memory and are believed to play a role in the connection of scent to particular memories.

Parahippocampal Gyrus

As you might suspect from its name, the parahippocampal gyrus surrounds the hippocampus. It plays an important role in memory encoding and retrieval and in the recognition of environmental scenes (landscapes, rooms, and spaces rather than faces).

Cingulate Gyrus (Cortex)

A gyrus, according to the dictionary, is a "convoluted ridge between anatomical grooves." The cingulate gyrus is an encircling ridge that covers the corpus collosum. It helps the brain regulate emotions and pain and is involved in the fear response and the prediction (and avoidance) of negative consequences.

Septal Nuclei

The septal nuclei are a set of structures situated at the base of the forebrain with reciprocal neural connections to the olfactory bulbs, hippocampi, amygdalae, hypothalami, and thalami. Though they have no role in odor detection, these nuclei are thought to play a role in the brain's reward systems (reward-based cognitive processes) and emotional behaviors.

Nucleus Accumbens

Also in the basal forebrain, the nucleus accumbens is involved in reward and reinforcement learning, pleasure (including laughter), maternal behavior, addiction, impulsivity, aggression, and fear. It is also thought to play a role in the so-called placebo effect.

Pituitary Gland

The pituitary gland, considered the master endocrine gland, is located just below the thalamus and between the hypothalamus and pineal gland (a small endorcrine gland), and is functionally connected to the hypothalamus via the pituitary stalk. In spite of this interface, the pituitary gland does not form part of the limbic system. However, when we experience emotions—for example, joy or fear—these feelings cause the hypothalamus to signal the pituitary gland to release hormones that may affect blood pressure, stimulate the heart, and so on. In this way the pituitary carries out the directives of the limbic system. The pituitary gland is directly involved with metabolic and physiological hormone-induced functions and processes, such as growth, regulation of blood pressure, sex organ function, thyroid gland function, water balance via the kidneys, temperature control, pain relief, and the metabolic conversion of food into energy.

Trigeminal Nerve Receptors

The trigeminal nerve is the largest of the cranial nerves and extends in three twinned nerve branches across either side of the cranium and facial areas:

1. The **ophthalmic nerve** relays sensory information from the scalp, forehead, upper eyelid, conjunctiva and cornea of the eye, nose, nasal mucosa, frontal sinuses, and parts of the meninges.
2. The **maxillary nerve** relays sensory information from the lower eyelid, cheek, nares (openings of the nasal cavities), upper lip, upper teeth and gums, nasal mucosa, palate, roof of the pharynx, maxilla, ethmoid and sphenoid tissue, and parts of the meninges.
3. The **mandibular nerve** relays sensory information from the lower lip, lower teeth and gums, chin, jaw, parts of the external ear, and parts of the meninges and the mouth.

Trigeminal nerve receptors that extend into the olfactory epithelium, nasal cavity, mouth, and eyes detect sensations of pressure, pain, and temperature. Chemicals (including essential oils) that stimulate the trigeminal nerve receptors in the nose and throat produce sensations that might be described as hot, cold, tingling, or even irritating (menthol, for example, found in mint essential oil, produces feelings of cold at moderate concentration but feelings of heat at high concentration). Trigeminal nerve receptors add sensation to the experiential dynamics of odor perception, whether subtle or obvious, and play a role in the complex process of odor detection, identification, and consequential neuro-physio-psycho-emotional stimulation. Around 70 percent of all odorants stimulate the trigeminal nerve receptors (Leffingwell 2002).

The Olfactory Experience of Essential Oils

An essential oil comprises a complex mixture of about two hundred chemical components, and sometimes more. Though researchers have identified most of these chemical components, and though essential oils have a fairly predictable chemical profile, there remain many variables that influence the human response to any specific essential oil.

To begin, essential oils naturally vary in composition depending on the particularities of the plants they are extracted from: the subspecies or variety of the plants, where they grew, growing conditions in that year, and how the plants were harvested, among other factors. Chemical variance (and therefore odor profile and quality) can occur between essential oils extracted from plants from the same botanical species that are grown in different regions, and even between essential oils extracted from the same plants if they are harvested more than once—for example, from a crop yielding flowers or fruits in early spring and then again in late summer. Consequently, each individual specimen of essential oil demonstrates a unique, multidynamic chemical and odor character or "fingerprint" according to the presence, quantity, and combination of its various constituents (these variations are expected to fall within a specified range).

Furthermore, despite all that we know and can predict about an essential oil's chemical profile and how those constituents affect the body, our first response to a scent is usually subjective. Our perception, psycho-emotional-physiological state, and environmental context add further dynamics. In other words, our physiological homeostatic chemical balance, state of health, gender, mood, personal likes and dislikes, memories, and sense of anticipation and expectation, along with the time of day, month, year, season, and environment, are influential factors that play a role in how we respond to an odor at any given time.

Structures within the limbic system engage multilaterally, instantly generating a complex cluster of interactive psycho-emotional, physiological, and behavioral responses. Thus, it is difficult to absolutely attribute, beyond general indication, specific psycho-emotional actions to particular essential oils. Likewise, it is difficult to solely attribute such actions to one specific brain region, hormone, or function; there are so many variables at play, and they are virtually impossible to disentangle from one another.

Essential oils are, consequently, generally therapeutically classified under umbrella terms such as stimulating, sedating, restorative, and so on. However, many essential oils actually possess both stimulating and sedating properties (for example, bergamot, chamomile, clary sage, geranium, lavender, marjoram, patchouli, and ylang ylang), while others are more sedating/less stimulating or more stimulating/less sedating, rather than being purely one or the other.

The subjective terms used to describe the psycho-emotional effects of essential oils generally fall into three categories: stimulating, harmonizing, and soothing.

Stimulating Effects	Harmonizing Effects	Soothing Effects
Invigorating	Balancing	Calming
Refreshing	Restorative	Grounding
Strengthening		Sedating
Uplifting		Warming

Once absorbed by the body, essential oils appear to work in a targeted manner to support or restore physical and psycho-emotional balance, stimulate the immune system, and act against pathogens. In their book *Aromatherapy: Scent and Psyche,* aromatherapists Peter and Kate Damian suggest that, due to the their natural design, essential oils act to instigate a contralateral response that harmonizes both brain hemispheres, instigating at one and the same time psychological, psychosomatic, and physiological responses. They refer to essential oils as "nature's optimal scents," stating that they are psychoactively more quickly effective, even in small doses, than synthetic fragrances, perfumes, and aromas, when absorbed via inhalation (Damian 1995, 149).

The Blood-Brain Barrier

The blood-brain barrier (BBB) is a highly selective barrier designed to protect the brain from infiltration by neurotoxins and pathogenic bacteria. The BBB keeps blood and other circulatory fluids separate from the brain's intracellular fluid and also helps maintain the consistent chemical balance necessary to support the brain's neurological functioning by acting as a very controlled filtration system.

In most of the body, capillaries are lined with endothelial tissues whose cells are spaced far enough apart to allow the passage of substances into and out of the capillaries. In contrast, the endothelial cells lining the capillaries in the BBB are densely connected, with closer, more tightly knit junctions. Astrocyte cells surround the brain's capillaries like a sleeve, perhaps contributing to the BBB's controlled permeability.

The BBB allows only highly selective passage (by passive diffusion) of water, oxygen, some gases, and certain molecules, such as amino acids and glucose, that are vital for neural function. Lipophilic essential oil constituents are among those able to penetrate the BBB, and thus they are able to interact with various receptor sites in the brain, such as those for gamma-aminobutyric acid (GABA) and glutamate (Tisserand and Young 2014, 51).

Indeed, there are numerous studies (mainly conducted by or on behalf of the food and manufacturing, cosmetic and pharmaceutical industries) exploring the psychotherapeutic effects of essential oils on attention, concentration, productivity, mental-emotional stimulation and sedation, mood states (anxiety, depression, agitation, restlessness), memory, and insomnia. Studies using animals, such as mice, although ethically controversial, eliminate many potentially influential subjective psycho-emotional variables when exploring the basic physiological and behavioral effects of essential oils and provide very useful indications. However, these studies do not completely reflect the complexities of real-life scenarios when applied to humans, where the idiosyncratic psycho-emotional and hedonistic responses to essential oils contribute to the outcome of their actions or, conversely, the complex influence that essential oils actually have on the individual's psyche, cognition, and physiological function (the inside-out, outside-in response).

The brain is responsive to external sensory input and neurological stimulation and facilitates internal homeostasis, environmental awareness, consciousness of a deeper sense of being, and relationships with other people and the external world. Fragrance detection triggers numerous neurological, physiological, emotional, and hedonistic responses at the same time, and they are difficult to disentangle. While it may be very difficult to prove or explain specifically how essential oils affect the brain, their vaporizing odorous molecules do instigate (to varying degrees) neurological responses that appear to affect mood, emotion, memory, perception, concentration, and cognition (either via inhalation or circulatory absorption), even if this influence is only temporary. Meanwhile, research and deliberation continue in a quest for better understanding.

The Olfactory Response and Memory

Scent memory is more tenacious compared with other senses (sight, touch, hearing). Memory is reinforced and enhanced and may last or linger longer when multiple sensory stimulations occur at the same time. This is especially the case when less consciously controlled cognitive processes—those that do not involve judgment, deliberation, reasoning, or rational evaluation—are being performed, such as creative tasks, learning or performing by rote, and so on (this works the same for negative and positive experiences). Thus, activities such as massage, meditation, visualization, or relaxation techniques may be positively enhanced and experientially memorably reinforced in our memory when complementary essential oils are vaporized at the same time (and vice versa).

Neuroscientist Rachel Herz is an expert on the psychological science of smell. While exploring the role of odor-evoked memories, she significantly observed that any scent that evokes a happy autobiographical memory for a given individual has the potential to increase positive emotions, decrease negative moods, lower stress, and decrease inflammatory immune responses. She also found that odor-evoked memories may

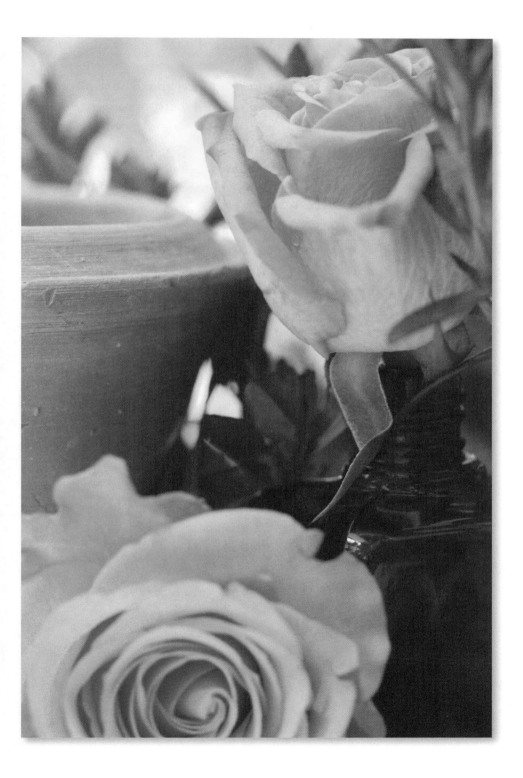

stimulate specific emotions, such as self-confidence, motivation, and vigor. Herz found that memories elicited by odors are more emotionally potent than memories evoked by other sensory stimuli, and when a salient emotion is experienced during odor exposure, the effectiveness of the resulting odor memory cue is enhanced, illustrated through observed increase in activity in the amygdala (Herz 2016, 22).

In a 2000 study on the effects of aromatherapy on children with learning difficulties, Vicki Pitman (herbalist, aromatherapist, reflexologist and author of *Aromatherapy: A Practical Approach,* among other works) exploited this salient connection between scent and memory to help hyperactive children manage their restlessness. She asked the children to use visualization and self-massage during exposure to selected essential oils to instill a sense of calmness and peace that they could later recall and experience when deliberately inhaling the scent of the same essential oil(s) as a memory cue, applied and used to calm their behavior and assist them in focusing on tasks. As a result, she observed that in combination, essential oils and relaxation techniques did improve students' concentration and ability to remain calm longer and to recover quickly from upsets.

LIMBIC SYSTEM STRUCTURES AND ESSENTIAL OILS THAT STRONGLY INFLUENCE THEM

In spite of the complexities observed previously, certain essential oils, due to their characteristic profile, appear to have an affinity for certain structures in the limbic system. The essential oils listed below are those that may potentially have the most pronounced effect on the associated limbic system structure. Serenity Essential Oils are indicated in boldface.

LIMBIC SYSTEM STRUCTURE	ESSENTIAL OILS WITH POTENTIALLY STRONG INFLUENCE
Pituitary gland (via the hypothalamus)	Clary sage *(Salvia sclarea)*
	Jasmine *(Jasminum officinale)*
	Patchouli *(Pogostemon cablin)*
	Rose otto *(Rosa × centifolia, R. × damascena)*
	Ylang ylang *(Cananga odorata)*

LIMBIC SYSTEM STRUCTURE	ESSENTIAL OILS WITH POTENTIALLY STRONG INFLUENCE
Hypothalamus	Bergamot *(Citrus bergamia)*
	Frankincense *(Boswellia carterii, B. sacra)*
	Geranium *(Pelargonium graveolens, P. × asperum)*
	Rosewood *(Aniba rosaeodora)*
Anterior thalamic nuclei	Clary sage *(Salvia sclarea)*
	Grapefruit *(Citrus paradisi)*
	Jasmine *(Jasminum officinale)*
	Rose otto *(Rosa × centifolia, R. × damascena)*
Amygdala	Black pepper *(Piper nigrum)*
	Geranium *(Pelargonium graveolens, P. × asperum)*
	Lemon *(Citrus limon)*
	Melissa *(Melissa officinalis)*
	Peppermint *(Mentha × piperita)*
	Rosemary *(Rosmarinus officinalis)*
	Thyme *(Thymus vulgaris)*
Hippocampus	Black pepper *(Piper nigrum)*
	Geranium *(Pelargonium graveolens, P. × asperum)*
	Lemon *(Citrus limon)*
	Melissa *(Melissa officinalis)*
	Peppermint *(Mentha × piperita)*
	Rosemary *(Rosmarinus officinalis)*
	Thyme *(Thymus vulgaris)*

**Psycho-emotional Conditions
That Essential Oils May Ease**

Anger

Anxiety

Depression

Fear

Grief

Headaches

Insomnia

Mental fog

Mental exhaustion

Mood swings

Nervous exhaustion

Nervous tension

Restlessness

Shock

THE PSYCHO-EMOTIONAL/LIMBIC
INFLUENCE OF SERENITY ESSENTIAL OILS

ESSENTIAL OIL	POTENTIAL CHARACTERISTIC PSYCHO-EMOTIONAL ACTION AND SUPPORT	POTENTIAL ASSOCIATED LIMBIC STRUCTURE
Cajeput (*Melaleuca cajuputi*)	Aids concentration, clears and stimulates the mind and thoughts, eases apathy, fosters courage in finding new pathways and managing change, strengthens resolve and spirit	Anterior thalamic nuclei
Carrot seed (*Daucus carota*)	Eases anxiety, apathy, indecisiveness, mental and emotional exhaustion, and mental fog; calms experience of stress and confusion; helps with inability to move on; revitalizing; nervous system sedative	Anterior thalamic nuclei and hypothalamus

ESSENTIAL OIL	POTENTIAL CHARACTERISTIC PSYCHO-EMOTIONAL ACTION AND SUPPORT	POTENTIAL ASSOCIATED LIMBIC STRUCTURE
Chamomile, German (*Matricaria recutita*)	Eases agitation, anxiety, depression/low mood, headaches, hypersensitivity, impatience, insomnia, irritability/intolerance, migraine, mood swings, nervous tension, and premenstrual tension; calms experience of stress; mental (calms an active mind) and nervous system sedative	Anterior thalamic nuclei and hypothalamus
Chamomile, Roman (*Anthemis nobilis*)	Eases agitation, anger, anxiety, depression/low mood, fear, hyperactivity, hypersensitivity, impatience, insomnia, irritability, panic attacks, premenstrual tension, restlessness, and solar plexus tension; calms experience of stress; mental, emotional, and nervous system sedative	Anterior thalamic nuclei, hypothalamus, and amygdala
Cypress (*Cupressus sempervirens*)	Eases anger, anxiety, confusion and indecisiveness, fear/paranoia, grief, impatience, inability to concentrate, irritability, nervous tension, premenstrual tension, stress, stress-related conditions, and uncontrollable crying; helps with inability to move on or to stop dwelling on unpleasant events; regulates autonomic nervous system; sedative	Anterior thalamic nuclei, hypothalamus, amygdala, and hippocampus
Frankincense (*Boswellia carterii, B. sacra*)	Eases anger, anxiety, confusion and indecisiveness, depression and low mood, fear and paranoia, grief, hyperactivity, impatience, irritability and intolerance, mood swings, nervous tension, panic attacks (calms and relaxes breathing), premenstrual tension, resentment and disappointment, and sadness and despair; helps with inability to move on, to stop dwelling on unpleasant events, or to let go of unwanted thoughts and memories; sedative; supports meditation and finding inner tranquillity	Anterior thalamic nuclei, hypothalamus, amygdala, and hippocampus
Galbanum (*Ferula galbaniflua*)	Balancing; both sedative and stimulant; calms erratic moods, nervous tension, menopausal symptoms, premenstrual tension, stress, and stress-related conditions; tonic; lifts mood and is restorative (nerves)	Hypothalamus

THE PSYCHO-EMOTIONAL/LIMBIC
INFLUENCE OF SERENITY ESSENTIAL OILS (*continued*)

ESSENTIAL OIL	POTENTIAL CHARACTERISTIC PSYCHO-EMOTIONAL ACTION AND SUPPORT	POTENTIAL ASSOCIATED LIMBIC STRUCTURE
Geranium *(Pelargonium graveolens, P. × asperum)*	Both sedative and stimulant; eases anxiety, depression and low mood, headaches, jealousy, nervous tension, menopausal symptoms, mood swings, premenstrual tension, stress, and stress-related conditions; balances the nerves and solar plexus; uplifting; endocrine stimulant (hormonelike)	Anterior thalamic nuclei, hypothalamus, amygdala, and hippocampus
Lavender, English and spike *(Lavandula angustifolia, L. latifolia)*	Sedative at low dosages, stimulant at high dosages; eases agitation, anger, anxiety, depression, grief, headaches, insomnia, irritability, manic depression (professional support required), mood swings, nervous tension, panic, premenstrual tension, sense of hopelessness, shock, solar plexus tension, stress, stress-related conditions, and suspiciousness	Anterior thalamic nuclei, hypothalamus, and amygdala
Mandarin *(Citrus reticulata)*	Awakens; brings out the inner child; good for quelling anxiety, depression and low mood, hyperactivity (although orange can encourage hyperactivity, mandarin is calming), insomnia, nervous tension, panic attacks, premenstrual tension, restlessness, stress, and stress-related conditions; has a sedative quality	Hypothalamus and amygdala
Patchouli *(Pogostemon cablin)*	Sedative at low dosages, stimulant at high dosages; eases apathy, confusion and indecisiveness, depression and low mood, nervous exhaustion, nervous tension, panic attacks, premenstrual tension, stress, and stress-related conditions; endocrine stimulant; supports meditation and a sense of spirituality	Anterior thalamic nuclei, hypothalamus, and pituitary (via the hypothalamus)
Petitgrain *(Citrus aurantium var. amara)*	Eases anger, anxiety, depression, hyperactivity, insomnia, mental fog, nervous exhaustion, nervous tension, premenstrual tension, sense of hopelessness, stress, and stress-related conditions; nervous system sedative	Hypothalamus and amygdala

ESSENTIAL OIL	POTENTIAL CHARACTERISTIC PSYCHO-EMOTIONAL ACTION AND SUPPORT	POTENTIAL ASSOCIATED LIMBIC STRUCTURE
Rose otto *(Rosa × damascena, Rosa × centifolia)*	Sedative at low dosages, stimulant at high dosages; eases agitation, anger, anxiety, depression (especially postnatal) and low mood, fear and paranoia, grief (and sense of loss), hatred, headaches (tension and hormonal), hypersensitivity, insomnia, jealousy, migraine, nervous tension, panic attacks, premenstrual tension, resentment and disappointment, sadness and despair, stress, and stress-related conditions; endocrine stimulant (hormonelike); aphrodisiac	Anterior thalamic nuclei, hypothalamus, amygdala, and pituitary (via the hypothalamus)
Spikenard *(Nardostachys jatamansi, N. grandiflora)*	Balances sympathetic nervous system with parasympathetic nervous system (tonic to the sympathetic nervous system, regulates the parasympathetic nervous system); grounding; eases anxiety, grief, hatred, headaches and migraine, hyperactivity, hysteria, impatience, insomnia, irritability, menopausal symptoms, nervous indigestion, nervous tension, panic attacks, premenstrual syndrome (PMS), restlessness, stress, and stress-related conditions; sedative	Anterior thalamic nuclei and hypothalamus
Tea tree *(Melaleuca alternifolia)*	Revitalizing and stimulating; cleansing; helpful for apathy, nervous exhaustion, and shock	Anterior thalamic nuclei and hypothalamus
Vetivert *(Vetiveria zizanioides)*	Reduces symptoms of withdrawal for someone coming off medication (especially tranquilizers); eases anxiety, confusion and indecisiveness, debility, depression, hyperactivity, hypersensitivity, impatience, insomnia, menopausal symptoms, mental exhaustion, nervous tension, panic attacks, premenstrual tension, stress, and stress-related conditions; encourages feelings of tranquillity; sedative to the nervous system; grounding	Anterior thalamic nuclei, hypothalamus, and amygdala

Odor Receptors

Odor receptors are found in many tissues, not just the olfactory epithelium. They exist throughout the body in organ tissue (for example, the liver, heart, kidneys, spleen, colon, lungs, brain, and testes) and epidermal tissue, and they are able to detect a multitude of compounds. Just as in olfactory detection, odor receptors in other parts of the body detect odor molecules (using the same lock-and-key mechanism) and in turn trigger and relay neural signals, which activate a cellular response. For example, odor receptors in the kidneys help control metabolic function and regulate blood pressure. Odor receptors within the testes aid fertilization through attraction, guiding the sperm cell to the ovulated egg. Keratinocytes, the major cells of the epidermis, contain olfactory receptors; odor molecules stimulate these cells, affecting cell proliferation, migration, regeneration, and rejuvenation—a significant process in wound healing. The discovery of the existence of odor receptors beyond the olfactory epithelium, however, is relatively recent, and further research is required to ascertain the extent of the function of these cells. Nonetheless, this discovery can help explain the healing, regenerating, and rejuvenating properties, among others, of essential oils (Busse et al 2014; Stone 2014; Griffin, Kafadar, and Pavlath 2009; Pluznick et al. 2008; Spehr et al. 2003).

The Respiratory Response to Essential Oils

Passing through the nose and across the olfactory epithelium, oxygen-rich air containing essential oil molecules continues its journey down the trachea (wind pipe), into the bronchi (tubes entering the lungs), and then into the lung cavity, where gaseous exchange takes place, facilitated by the alveoli. The alveoli are tiny specialized hollow air sacs found at the end of alveolar ducts and atria located at the tip of the bronchioles, which branch from the bronchi. Imagine a tree trunk (trachea) that branches into two (bronchi), each producing smaller branches and twigs (bronchioles) that spread into each lung, and the alveoli are the leaves. Each lung contains around 350 million alveoli, which collectively provide approximately 70 to 100 square meters of surface area. The thin porous membrane surrounding each alveolus contains a matrix, or network, of pulmonary arterial and venous capillaries, which facilitate the movement of oxygen and carbon dioxide between air and blood.

Oxygen, along with other airborne molecules, such as those from essential oils, diffuses from the inhaled air momentarily contained within the lungs into arterial capillaries, from where the oxygen-infused blood travels away from the lungs (through arterioles and arteries) via the circulatory system to cells throughout the body; thus essential oil molecules are carried via the blood into the internal organs and cells. The cells in exchange release carbon dioxide (CO_2) into the blood, which is carried from organs and other tissues via veins and ultimately into alveolar venous capillaries. There, along with other blood-borne volatile compounds, CO_2 diffuses out through the thin porous membrane surface into the air still held momentarily within the lungs, before being excreted from the body via exhalation of the breath.

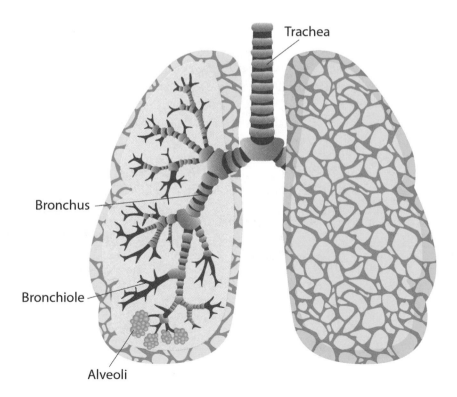

The lungs

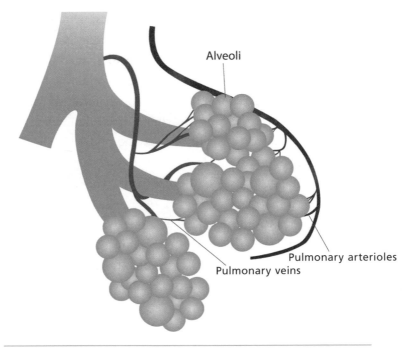

Alveoli

Pulmonary arterioles

Pulmonary veins

Pulmonary arterioles carry deoxygenated blood from the heart to the lungs, and pulmonary veins return oxygenated blood to the heart. (This is the exception to the usual rule—pulmonary arteries are the only arteries in the body that carry deoxygenated blood, and the pulmonary veins are the only veins that carry oxygenated blood.)

SERENITY ESSENTIAL OILS
AND THEIR RESPIRATORY EFFECTS

ESSENTIAL OIL	ACTIONS	RESPIRATORY CONDITIONS THAT MAY BENEFIT
Cajeput (*Melaleuca cajuputi*)	Analgesic (mild), antimicrobial, antispasmodic, antiseptic, expectorant, mucolytic	Asthma, bronchitis, catarrh, colds, coughs, flu, hay fever, laryngitis, pain (inflammation, muscular spasm, congestion), sinusitis, sore throat, upper respiratory tract infections
Carrot seed (*Daucus carota*)	Anti-inflammatory, smooth muscle relaxant	Bronchitis, chronic pulmonary problems, coughs; strengthens mucous membranes

ESSENTIAL OIL	ACTIONS	RESPIRATORY CONDITIONS THAT MAY BENEFIT
Chamomile, German (*Matricaria recutita*)	Antiallergenic, anti-inflammatory, antispasmodic, bactericidal	Asthma, catarrh, hay fever, mouth ulcers, teething, tonsillitis
Chamomile, Roman (*Anthemis nobilis*)	Analgesic, antiseptic, antispasmodic, bactericidal	Asthma (especially nervous), mouth ulcers, teething
Cypress (*Cupressus sempervirens*)	Anti-inflammatory, antispasmodic, antitussive, mucolytic	Asthma, bronchitis, colds, flu, hoarseness, laryngitis, pain (inflammation, muscular spasm, congestion), pulmonary infections, sinusitis, spasmodic cough, sore throat, upper respiratory tract infections, whooping cough
Frankincense (*Boswellia carterii, B. sacra*)	Anti-inflammatory, antiseptic, expectorant	Asthma, bronchitis, catarrh, colds, coughs, flu, laryngitis, panic attacks (calms and relaxes breathing), sore throat, upper respiratory tract infections; eases shortness of breath and encourages deep breathing
Galbanum (*Ferula galbaniflua*)	Analgesic, anti-inflammatory, antimicrobial, antispasmodic, decongestant, expectorant	Asthma, bronchial spasms, catarrh, chronic coughs, mucous congestion
Geranium (*Pelargonium graveolens, P. × asperum*)	Anti-inflammatory, antiseptic	Asthma, colds, catarrh, pulmonary infection and viruses, sore throat, tonsillitis
Lavender, English (*Lavandula angustifolia*)	Analgesic, anti-inflammatory, antimicrobial, antispasmodic	Asthma, bronchitis, catarrh, colds, flu, gingivitis, halitosis, hay fever, laryngitis, pulmonary infections and viruses; relaxes and eases breathing (panic attacks)
Lavender, spike (*Lavandula latifolia*)	Anti-inflammatory, mucolytic	Asthma, bronchitis, hay fever, laryngitis, sinusitis, tonsillitis
Mandarin (*Citrus reticulata*)	Antiseptic, antispasmodic	Asthma, bronchitis, coughs

SERENITY ESSENTIAL OILS
AND THEIR RESPIRATORY EFFECTS (*continued*)

ESSENTIAL OIL	ACTIONS	RESPIRATORY CONDITIONS THAT MAY BENEFIT
Patchouli (*Pogostemon cablin*)	Anti-inflammatory, anti-microbial, antiseptic, anti-viral, bactericidal	Panic attacks and shortness of breath due to anxiety (calms the flow of breathing); respiratory infections
Petitgrain (*Citrus aurantium* var. *amara*)	Anti-inflammatory, antiseptic, antispasmodic	Asthma (nervous), colds, flu, hay fever, respiratory infections; eases labored breathing and stress-related shallow breathing
Rose Otto (*Rosa × damascena, Rosa × centifolia*)	Anti-inflammatory, antiseptic, antispasmodic, antiviral, bactericidal.	Chronic asthma, coughs, hay fever, mouth ulcers, sore throat
Spikenard (*Nardostachys jatamansi, N. grandiflora*)	Anti-infectious, anti-inflammatory, bactericidal, fungicidal	Oral candida, panic attacks (calms the flow of breathing through psycho-emotional influence), respiratory infections, and sore throats.
Tea tree (*Melaleuca alternifolia*)	Anti-inflammatory, antimicrobial, antispasmodic, antiviral, bactericidal, expectorant, immune stimulant	Asthma, bronchitis, catarrh, colds, coughs, ENT (ear, nose, and throat) infections, gum disease, hay fever, mycosis, sinusitis, sore throat, tonsillitis, upper respiratory tract infections
Vetivert (*Vetiveria zizanioides*)	Antiseptic, antispasmodic	Panic attacks; deepens and regulates breathing

Note: Asthma is one of the respiratory conditions that can benefit from essential oil therapy, but do **not** use essential oils during an asthma attack. For treatment of asthma as a chronic condition (not during an attack), use essential oils topically at a very low dose (0.5 to 1% dilution).

Adverse Effects of Airborne Substances

Airborne molecules evaporating from fresh, appropriately stored essential oils rarely cause adverse effects. However, old, oxidized essential oils—especially herbaceaous oils and those with high terpene content—may instigate a negative reaction. Chemically extracted absolutes contain residues of the solvent applied to soak out the oils from the plant material and may also instigate an adverse reaction; absolutes are not classified as "pure essential oils." If you are already allergic or intolerant or sensitive to certain chemicals and substances found in household products, perfumes, air fresheners, foods, metals, et cetera, you may be predisposed to react adversely to certain molecules found in essential oils.

The two principal adverse effects of airborne ambient essential oils and other inhaled substances are bronchial hyperreactivity (excessive contraction of the bronchioles and small airways) and sensory irritation, which includes both eye and airway irritation. Sensory irritation is a nonallergic response, although it can exacerbate preexisting and undetected allergic conditions. Bronchial hyperactivity can be an allergic or nonallergic response, and it may be associated with respiratory disease such as asthma, allergic rhinitis, or chronic obstructive pulmonary disease (COPD).

There are many potential contributors to irritation caused by airborne substances, which makes it difficult to differentiate a single causative factor. They may include, for example, chemicals within air fresheners, hair sprays, cleaning products, exhaust fumes, industrial emissions, oxidized terpenes, and toxic substances such as chloroform, formaldehyde, acetaldehyde, benzene, toluene, xylene, and styrene. Pain receptors and the trigeminal nerves (see pages 32–33) are responsive to irritants; warning symptoms may include irritation, tickling, burning, warming, cooling, or stinging in the nasal and oral cavities, sinuses, and eyes (Tisserand and Young 2014, 100).

Methods of Application for Olfactory Absorption

PRIMARY

Tissue or smelling strip

Steam inhalation

Perfume

Facial products—creams, lotions, gels, or oils

SECONDARY (EXUDING VAPORS)

Massage with oil

Environmental diffuser

Candle-lit resin burner

Incense

Body lotions and oils

Bath oils

Shower diffusion (vaporized in steam)

OTHER SOURCES

Foods/herbs/spices

Household products

PERCUTANEOUS (SKIN) ABSORPTION

The skin is the largest organ of the body and, along with its functional structures (sweat glands, hair follicles, capillaries, et cetera), forms part of the integumentary system. Its function is to contain and protect muscles, bones, ligaments, and internal organs from damage and to prevent excessive loss of water and vital nutrients. It provides a semi-porous barrier that selectively manages the infiltration and excretion of substances to and from the body and facilitates insulation, temperature regulation (through shivering and perspiration), release of enzymes and other waste products of metabolism (a process of detoxification, again through perspiration), and the initiation of certain immune mechanisms (for example, through the antigen activity of Langerhans cells, which are embedded in the skin). Skin also protects the body from invading bacteria, viruses, and other potential contaminants. (For example, sebum, released by the sebaceous glands, when combined with sweat creates a fine acid film on the skin's surface, known as the acid mantle, which acts as a protective barrier and prevents water loss.) Skin comprises three layers:

+ **The epidermis** (outer layer), which consists of dead epidermal cells embedded in a lipid matrix responsible for reducing permeability to water.
+ **The dermis,** which contains blood and lymph vessels, nerves, sweat and sebaceous glands, and hair follicles.
+ **The subcutaneous layer,** which consists primarily of fat.

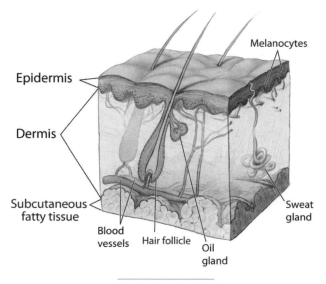

Layers of the skin

The stratum corneum, the most superficial layer of the skin (see diagram on page 12), comprises a matrix of both hydrophilic (water-loving) and lipophilic (fat- or oil-loving) cells and regions and provides a very effective barrier. Only very small molecules are able to penetrate the stratum corneum and then only under certain conditions. Essential oils consist of a mixture of various chemical molecules. Once applied to the skin, essential oil molecules separate and disperse across, and into, the stratum corneum, diffusing and permeating via different pathways according to their polar and nonpolar bonding behaviors. Diffusion is facilitated via four routes:

1. Paracellular (intercellular)—*between* skin cells
2. Transcellular—*through* skin cells
3. Hair follicles and sebaceous ducts (bypassing the stratum corneum), assisted by the presence of sebum, the oily secretion of the sebaceous glands that waterproofs and lubricates the hair and skin
4. Sweat glands

Less than 10 percent of the essential oil applied to the superficial layers of the skin actually passes, via capillaries embedded within the dermis, into the circulatory system (Tisserand and Young 2014, 42). Due to their highly volatile nature, many essential oil molecules evaporate from the skin's warm surface into the surrounding atmosphere; some of these potentially find their way into the body via inhalation. Those molecules that do not pass through the skin and do not immediately evaporate remain suspended within the epidermis. Some of these molecules may linger for up to seventy-two hours. Most of the molecules able to diffuse into the dermis, however, usually do so within the first twenty-four hours. Others irreversibly bind to cutaneous proteins (such as keratin), are metabolized by cutaneous enzymes, or gradually evaporate.

Carrier mediums such as creams, lotions, and vegetable oils can enhance permeability, reduce essential oil evaporation, and reduce the irritant effect of many essential oils. Carrier mediums act as an emollient vehicle to disperse essential oils across the skin's surface. Vegetable oils create a barrier that prevents water loss and slows essential oil evaporation. Many vegetable oils also possess significant therapeutic qualities of their own that can enhance the skin-healing action of essential oils or quell certain potential irritant compounds (see the box on pages 56–59). The combination of vegetable oils, essential oils, and superficial and deep tissue stimulation through massage provides a potent therapeutic modality (remembering, too, that essential oils are also likely inhaled during this process, stimulating and further enhancing psycho-emotional and physiological responses and benefits).

Occlusion (covering, usually with a towel or sheet) of the skin area immediately after application of an essential oil further reduces evaporation and supports penetration of the essential oil molecules.

Carrier Mediums for Dermal Applications of Essential Oils

The carrier mediums here are among the most effective for blending with essential oils for application to the skin. In addition to being good carriers for essential oils, they provide their own benefits to the skin. See chapter 7 for information about how to blend essential oils with these carrier mediums in various formulations.

Vegetable/Plant Oils
Used for: Various skin conditions, especially dry skin.
Benefits: Nonirritant, moisturizing, skin softening, emollient. Barrier against water loss. Supports skin's acid mantle. Lubricating (useful in massage). Assists essential oil (especially lipophilic molecules) penetration into the epidermis.
Cautions: Leaves an oily film on skin. Short shelf life; will become rancid over time, especially if not stored correctly.
Storage: Keep cool, replace lids immediately and keep tightly secured to avoid oxidation, use within twelve months.
Note: Coconut oil contains saturated fat similar to that found in subcutaneous tissue, thus it penetrates the skin with ease. Its high acidic content aids the skin's pH balance and protects against bacteria invasion. Although coconut oil generally has a long shelf life, it can spoil if not stored correctly. (See Coconut entry in the following box.)

Creams
Viscous aqueous oil- or fat- (vegetable/plant) based emulsion
Used for: Dry or mature skin (dry skin—light cream; mature skin—rich cream). Facial skin care. Local/small area skin care.
Benefits: Cooling, emollient, moisturizing, and softening.
Cautions: Prone to bacterial and fungal contamination (due to water content).
Storage: Keep cool, replace lids immediately, and use within six weeks once opened or three months if stored unopened in a refrigerator.

Lotions

Similar in composition to cream but less viscous.

Used for: Dry to normal skin. Inflamed skin. Body and facial skin care.

Benefits: Soothing, cooling, refreshing, and moisturizing. Water in the lotion evaporates, providing a cooling effect.

Cautions: Prone to bacterial and fungal contamination (due to water content).

Storage: Keep cool, replace lids immediately, and use within six weeks once opened or three months if stored unopened in a refrigerator.

Ointments

Non-aqueous oil-, wax-, and/or plant-based thickening substance

Used for: Dry, scaly skin. First aid (antiseptic ointment). Local/small area skin care.

Benefits: Occlusive and emollient. Reduces loss of water from skin. Slows essential oil evaporation.

Cautions: Messy to apply (though ointments are generally used only in small amounts for first aid).

Storage: Keep cool, replace lids immediately, and use within four weeks if opened, three months if unopened and stored in a refrigerator.

Aloe Vera Gel

Used for: Exudative and acutely inflamed skin. Wounds. Facial skin care. Local/small area skin care.

Benefits: Cooling, soothing, and drying.

Cautions: May sting inflamed skin. Slightly sticky initially, but penetrating and drying to the skin.

Storage: Keep cool, replace lids immediately, and use within three months.

Honey

Used for: Facial skin care. Wounds, burns, ulcerated conditions.

Benefits: Clears infection. Antimicrobial. Promotes clean, healthy granulation of the skin tissue.

Cautions: Sticky. Messy to apply.

Storage: Store in a cool, dry place and keep the lid tightly secured to avoid water or moisture contamination. Honey has an indefinite shelf life.

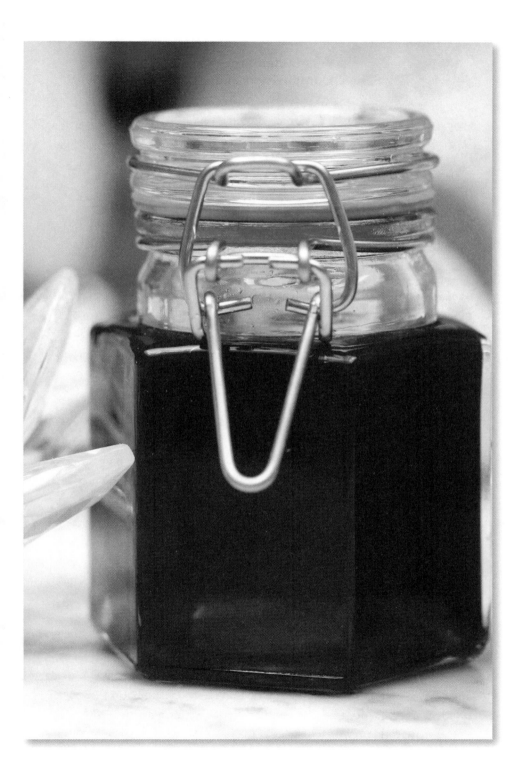

Vegetable/Plant Oils:
Their Composition and Qualities

This list is not exhaustive. However, the oils presented here provide a valuable range of qualities sufficient for most requirements. They can be applied singularly or can be blended together. Avocado is very viscous and benefits from being blended with a less viscous oil, such as grapeseed, when used for massage. Borage seed oil and jojoba oil can be expensive. Dilution "spreads" the cost when applying these in body massage or to large areas of skin. Undiluted, they are wonderful face oils, and can be applied to other small areas of skin. Recommended percentages are included below to guide dilution.

Avocado *(Persea americana, P. gratissima)*
Extraction: Cold pressed
Description: Dark, rich green to an emerald-green hue. Thick and viscous. Little odor. The color comes from high levels of chlorophylls and carotenoids. Highly penetrative. Long shelf life.
Constituents: Oleic acid (50–74%), linoleic acid (6–20%), palmitic acid (5–25%), palmitoleic acid (1–12%), stearic acid (up to 3%), linolenic acid (up to 3%), beta-carotene, vitamins E, A, B_1, B_2, and D
Dilution: Use 10% avocado oil in another carrier oil for massage or to apply to large areas of skin (for ease of application). Increase this percentage or apply undiluted (this oil is very viscous) for facial, dry, or damaged skin.
Uses: Recommended for dry, itchy, dehydrated, scaly, or aging skin. Penetrates epidermis. Promotes skin regeneration. Useful for eczema, psoriasis, burns, and other wounds. Antioxidant.

Borage *(Borago officinalis)*
Extraction: Cold pressed or CO_2 extraction
Description: Golden (orange to red). Slightly viscous. Medium to strong seed-like odor. Poor stability and thus a short shelf life; keep cool.
Constituents: Linoleic acid (35–45%), oleic acid (14–20%), palmitic acid (8–13%), eicosenoic acid (3–5%), stearic acid (2–6%), erucic acid (1–3%)
Dilution: Use 10% borage oil in another carrier oil for massage or to apply to large areas of skin. Apply undiluted for facial skin care.
Uses: Recommended for all types of skin. Improves elasticity of skin. Anti-

inflammatory. Useful for psoriasis, eczema, seborrheic dermatitis, premature aging of skin.

Note: The most effective skin-enhancing and anti-inflammatory action (especially for arthritis) comes with internal use of borage oil as a nutritional supplement.

Calendula *(Calendula officinalis)*

Extraction: Macerated (infused) or CO_2 extracted

Description: Deep orange. Macerated in olive, sweet almond, sunflower, or grapeseed oil. Light hint of marigold in addition to odor of the oil used for infusion.

Constituents: Linoleic acid (50–74%), oleic acid (14–39%), palmitic acid (5.0–7.6%), stearic acid (2.7–6.5%), arachidic acid (up to 1%), icosenoic acid (up to 1%), docosanoic acid (up to 1%), alpha linolenic acid (up to 0.3%), essential oils, carotenoid pigments.

Dilution: Use 5 to 15% in another carrier oil for massage or to apply to large areas of skin. Use undiluted for facial skin or wound care.

Uses: Recommended for wound healing and tissue repair/regeneration. Antiseptic, antimicrobial. Reduces swelling. Useful for chapped skin, cracked hands and feet, chilblains, cracked nipples in nursing (the oil is nontoxic to infants), burns, acne, impetigo, eczema, insect bites, and ulcers.

Coconut *(Cocos nucifera),* Virgin

Extraction: Cold pressed

Description: White. Solid at cold temperature, liquefying when the ambient temperature is warm. Sweet coconutty odor. Has a long shelf life but can spoil if not stored correctly. Water will spoil coconut oil. Keep the lid tightly secured to avoid oxidation and store in a cool, dark place.

Fractionated coconut oil (steam distilled or hydrolyzed to remove long-chain fatty acids) remains in a liquid state at any temperature. Some therapists prefer fractionated coconut oil because it is easier to blend with other oils and apply to large areas of skin during massage. Unfractionated, virgin coconut oil is preferable—remember, it will easily return to a liquid state at about 76°F.

Constituents: Lauric acid (45–53%), myristic acid (16–21%), palmitic acid (6–10%), caprinic acid (5–8%), caprylic acid (4–12%), oleic acid (4–10%), stearic acid (2–4%), linoleic acid (0.5–3%), capronic acid (up to 10%)

Dilution: Use undiluted or use 10–50% coconut oil in another carrier oil or skin care product (such as cream or lotion).

Uses: Suitable for all skin types, including mature skin. Supports healing and repair of tissues, including for cases of psoriasis, eczema, and dermatitis. Moisturizing; softens skin and helps relieve dryness and flaking. Reduces inflammation. Supports the natural chemical balance of the skin. Promotes healthy looking hair and complexion. Provides protection from damaging effects of ultraviolet radiation from the sun.

Grapeseed *(Vitis vinifera)*

Extraction: Cold pressed from the seeds

Description: *(Organic)* Deep green. Viscous. Strong, earthy seed-like odor. *(Refined)* Pale yellow to colorless. Virtually odorless, with a fine consistency preferred for massage. Very stable.

Constituents: *(Organic)* Linoleic acid (58–78%), oleic acid (10-28%), stearic acid (2–6%), linolenic acid (up to 2%)
(Refined) Linoleic acid (55–81%), oleic acid (12–33%), palmitic acid (5–11%), stearic acid (2–8%), linolenic acid (up to 1.5%), a small amount of vitamin E

Dilution: Use undiluted.

Uses: Recommended for all skin types. Promotes balanced moisturization of the skin. Penetrates the epidermis. Slightly astringent; good for oily skin and acne.

Jojoba *(Simmondsia chinensis)*

Extraction: Cold pressed from the seed (which contains liquid wax; it's not technically an oil)

Description: Golden yellow (unrefined) to virtually colorless (refined). Semisolid at room temperature; solid at colder temperatures. Unrefined jojoba oil has a slight nutty odor. The refined oil is virtually odorless. Very stable (longer shelf life than vegetable oils). The oil is not digestible so it is used only topically, and not in cooking.

Constituents: 11-eicosenoic acid (65–80%), erucic acid (10–20%), oleic acid (5–15%), lignocetric acid (5%), nervonic acid (1%), palmitic acid (3%), palmitoleic acid (1%), stearic acid (1%), behenic acid (0.5%), arachidic acid (0.5%)

Dilution: Use undiluted or use 10% jojoba in another carrier oil for massage, or in skin care products, such as creams or lotions.

Uses: Recommended for all skin types. Mimics sebum. Readily penetrates the epidermis. Softens and moisturizes the skin. Indicated for eczema and psoriasis. Anti-inflammatory; invaluable for dermatitis, arthritis, and swellings. Also useful for hair care; coats, protects, renews, and adds shine.

Olive *(Olea europaea)*, Extra Virgin

Extraction: Cold pressed from hard ripe olives; extra virgin oil comes from the first pressing.

Description: Darkish yellow green. Thick texture. Fruity-peppery, rich aroma.

Constituents: Oleic acid (56–85%), palmitic acid (7.5–20%), linoleic acid (3.5–20%), stearic acid (0.5–5%), linolenic acid (up to 1%), arachidic acid (up to 1%), eicosenoic acid (up to 0.7%)

Dilution: Use undiluted or use 50% olive oil in another carrier medium.

Uses: Recommended for mature and dry skin. Useful for seborrheic dermatitis, atopic dermatitis, acne, psoriasis, bruises, sprains, insect bites, arthritis, and dehydrated, sore, inflamed skin. Helps prevent stretch marks during pregnancy. Reduces itchiness of pruritus. Natural sun filter, screening out up to 20% of the sun's rays *(though it should not be used alone as sunscreen)*.

Note: Use only cold-pressed, extra-virgin olive oil.

Essential oils are predominantly more lipophilic than hydrophilic and tend to naturally move from aqueous (watery) to lipid (oily or fatty) environments. Fat-loving lipophilic constituents diffuse more readily and more extensively than water-loving hydrophilic constituents. To facilitate absorption, or diffusion, from the dermis into the blood circulation, however, essential oil molecules do need to possess both hydrophilic and lipophilic qualities (cells rely on water to facilitate diffusion and osmosis, and blood plasma, which constitutes 55 percent of the blood, consists mostly of water).

Some essential oil constituents, especially terpene molecules, readily interact with skin lipids in a manner that reduces their barrier function. In fact, terpenes are sometimes used with topical medications to enhance their absorption through the skin. Numerous studies have confirmed the efficacy of terpenes in enhancing the permeability of the skin and absorption of chemical compounds (Cal 2006; Prasanthi and Lakshmi 2012; Carpentieri-Rodrigues, Zanluchi, and Grebogi 2007).

Terpene Degradation

Terpenes are the basic building blocks of essential oils and are found in all essential oils to varying degrees. They are alkenes (unsaturated hydrocarbons containing a double bond), tend to have low toxicity, and are often used to counterbalance, or quench, the irritant effects of other more reactive compounds, such as aldehydes (the highly irritant effect of citral, an aldehyde found in lemons, for example, is quenched by the presence of terpenes, such as D-limonene and alpha-pinene, that coexist within the fruit). However, terpenes are highly volatile, rapidly oxidize, and degrade or transmute into other functional chemicals that can ultimately render them toxic and/or irritant to the skin and mucous membranes.

Francis and Bui (2015) tested the chemical composition of lemon (*Citrus limonum*, a.k.a. *Citrus limon*), sweet orange (*Citrus sinensis*), and tangerine (*Citrus reticulata*) essential oils before and after partial evaporation. They found that rapid oxidization of monoterpene hydrocarbons, especially those more volatile than limonene, rendered the residual content with a dramatically increased quantity of sensitizing components, increasing the propensity for sensitization and irritation, most especially in the case of *Citrus limon*, which contains relatively high levels of citral. Thus, essential oils with a high terpene content have a limited shelf life.

In addition to citrus fruits and citrusy plants, such as melissa *(Melissa officinalis)*, which contains the aldehydes citral and citronellal, potentially sensitizing terpenes and aldehydes are found in Pinaceae species, such as pine *(Pinus mugo* var. *pumilio* and to a lesser extent *Pinus sylvestris)*; in Cupressaceae species, such as cade juniper *(Juniperus oxycedrus)* and to a lesser extent cypress *(Cupressus sempervirens)*; and in *Melaleuca* species, such as tea tree *(Melaleuca alternifolia)* and to a lesser extent cajeput *(Melaleuca cajuputi)*.

Permeability characteristics of the skin vary between individuals and between different areas of the body. Absorption is potentially more readily facilitated in areas where the stratum corneum is thinner, where tissue is less dense and there is less body fat, and where the skin is broken or damaged. It is slower where tissue is more dense and there is more body fat.

FACILITATED ABSORPTION	SLOWER ABSORPTION
Forehead	Abdomen
Mucous membranes	Back
Palms of the hands	Buttocks
Scalp	Chest
Shoulders	Legs
Soles (arches) of the feet	Heels of the feet
Injured or inflamed skin	Heels (palm side) of the hands

Other factors influencing percutaneous absorption include:

+ The chemical composition of the essential oil and its hydrophilic and lipophilic qualities
+ The age, quality, and condition of the essential oil
+ The quantity of essential oil that is applied
+ The frequency of application
+ The carrier medium that is used (lotion, cream, vegetable/plant oil, ointment, et cetera; see chapter 7)
+ The synergistic, potentiating, additive, or antagonistic interactions between constituents within the essential oil and the carrier medium
+ The synergistic, potentiating, additive, or antagonistic interaction between the essential oil and carrier medium and the surrounding tissue cells
+ The pH balance, quality, integrity, hydration or moisture content, temperature, age, and general condition of the skin
+ The area of the body where the essential oil is applied
+ The method of application (massage, compress, ointment, et cetera)

Points to consider:

+ Inflammation and skin trauma (damage or disease) dramatically increase skin permeability. They also significantly increase the risk of localized skin reactions and consequential propensity for sensitization.

+ Alcohol (as a carrier medium or pretreatment cleanser) increases the permeation speed of essential oils. (This is one reason that alcohol is often used as a base medium for perfumes.)

+ Essential oils—especially those with a high terpene content—penetrate the dermis more rapidly, with increased risk of skin irritation and sensitization, when applied neat (undiluted) than when suspended in a (skin-protecting) vegetable/plant oil, lotion, or cream.

+ The risk of skin irritation and/or sensitization is greatly increased if the essential oil has oxidized (due to age or poor storage conditions).

+ The amount of essential oil used and the frequency of application have significant bearing on the propensity for sensitization, irritation, and allergic reactions.

+ Some essential oils have rubefacient qualities, meaning that they increase surface area blood flow, thus potentially boosting the speed of absorption but also, again, the propensity to cause irritation or sensitization.

+ Large molecules are absorbed more slowly than small molecules. However, small molecules evaporate more quickly and may be lost before they are able to penetrate the skin. On the other hand, some larger molecules are too large to penetrate at all.

+ Some essential oil molecules have quenching or calming effects that may counterbalance the irritant effect of other molecules.

Percutaneous application appears to be most effective when treating conditions relating to the superficial layers of the skin and local underlying tissue (muscles, joints). However, Kerr (2002) observed both physiological and psycho-emotional outcomes (healing, infection control, pain reduction, moisturization, and improved mental attitude) in a trial exploring the effectiveness of a selected blend of essential oils in wound care for the elderly. Kerr also noted that the anti-infectious and analgesic effects of the essential oils—German chamomile *(Matricaria recutita),* English lavender *(Lavandula angustifolia),* myrrh *(Commiphora myrrha),* and tea tree *(Melaleuca alternifolia)*—improved significantly when the ratio of essential oils to carrier medium (aloe vera) was increased from 5 percent to 9 or 12 percent. He concluded, "Essential oils are very effective in treating small to medium wounds, skin abrasions, excoriations, skin infections, and other topical health problems providing an appropriate concentration of essential oil is used."

Bensouilah and Buck (2006) point to the close connection between the nervous system and the skin and the consequential influence that emotional stress can have in "precipitating, aggravating, or prolonging many skin diseases" and "delaying skin barrier recovery." They then note that sedative essential oils (citing, in particular, Bulgarian rose [*Rosa damascena*] essential oil in this context) may exert a dual role (psycho-emotional and physiological) in managing stress-related, or stress-exacerbated, skin disorders such as psoriasis, eczema, and acne. Frankincense *(Boswellia carterii, B. sacra)* is another essential oil cited as potentially possessing a simultaneous psycho-emotional and physio-immunological capacity to exert a calming influence on stress and stress-related conditions, while at the same time demonstrating a regenerative effect on the integumentary system when applied topically (Holmes 1999a).

Tisserand (1997, 79) also acknowledges that essential oils have both physiological and psychological effects. "The former," he says, "acts directly on the physical organism, the latter acts, via the sense of smell, on the mind, which in turn may cause a physiological effect." He notes that the psychological effect is much less predictable than the physical and goes on to observe:

> One is reminded of the organic nature of essences, and of their ability to adapt, normalise, or balance rather than simply stimulate or sedate. Their action, as I have suggested, is more complex and subtle, because each essence has an affinity with certain parts of the

body, certain areas of the mind, and certain types of emotion. Just as someone with a "hard heart" may develop heart disease, or hardening of the arteries, so the essences which relieve the physical condition may also act on the mental state. (Tisserand 1997, 100)

The complex nature of an essential oil's chemical composition can be seen as a reflection of the body's interconnectedness. During development of the human embryo, the brain, the nervous system, the sense organs (including the lining of the nasal cavity, sinuses, and mouth), and the skin are derived from the ectoderm (the outermost layer of cells or tissue of the embryo). Tisserand (1997, 8) suggests that, due to this common origin, it is not unreasonable to assume that there remain close connection between these systems, and that consequently essential oils, or other products, applied to an area of the skin will also affect connected systems and organs, whether or not skin penetration takes place. Dr. James Oschman, biochemist and author of *Energy Medicine in Therapeutics and Human Performance,* apparently confirming this potential, suggests that interconnection exists between the body's whole system, connective tissue, and membrane proteins and the structural fabric of the cell and nucleus, which he collectively refers to as the living matrix. According to Oschman, messages are rapidly relayed throughout this matrix via a rippling effect between the cells that form fascia, which is the continuous membrane sheath that covers, separates, and therefore also touches the organs, vessels, and muscle tissue throughout the body. In this way, signals are relayed between local cells and distant cells and directly to the nervous system—thus, a whole-body response is initiated no matter where contact originally occurs. This may, in some way, explain the far-reaching effects of essential oils.

In terms of essential oil application, Buckle (2007, 86), on a cautionary note, found that "patients taking several medications at the same time are more likely to be sensitive to essential oils than patients who are not taking several medications," also noting that "those who have an allergy-like illness such as asthma, eczema, or hay fever may also be more sensitive to potential allergenic compounds, such as lactones, found in essential oils." (A person's reactivity to an essential oil also depends on the individual's idiosyncratic level of tolerance. As a precaution, patch testing essential oils and any carrier medium is recommended for those who are taking medication, who are prone to allergies and/or sensitivity, or who are recovering from acute or long-term illness. See the guidelines on page 96 for more information.)

Applied appropriately, essential oils and their spectrum of potentiating therapeutic qualities complementarily support the multidynamic functions of the integumentary system.

Water and Its Vital Role within the Body

Water is essential for life. All of the body's processes depend on water, from cellular osmosis and metabolic reaction to the transportation of nutrients and waste material to temperature regulation. Just 8 percent of the body's water requirements are met through biochemical processes in the body, which means that the remaining 92 percent must be consumed every day.

The body is approximately 60 percent water, which can be categorized into two types:

- **Intracellular** (within cells) fluid makes up around 67 percent (two-thirds) of the body's water. It contains moderate quantities of magnesium and sulfate ions and other solutes essential to electrolytic balance and healthy metabolism. It also constitutes part of the cellular matrix in which organelles are suspended and where chemical reactions take place.
- **Extracellular** (outside cells) fluid makes up around 26 percent of the body's water. It can be categorized as follow:

  - **Interstitial fluid** surrounds cells of a given tissue and maintains an environment conducive for the initiation of osmosis, supporting the movement of ions, proteins, and nutrients across the cell membrane, allowing a solute balance inside and outside the cell.
  - **Intravascular fluid** is primarily blood, which holds blood cells in suspension and also circulates colloids (globulins) and solutes (glucose and ions). Blood plasma, the pale yellow liquid component of blood, is 95 percent water and comprises around 7 percent of the body's water (and about 55 percent of the blood's volume). It

contains dissolved proteins, glucose, clotting factors, electrolytes, hormones, and carbon dioxide and serves as the protein reserve for the body. Another intravascular fluid is cerebrospinal fluid, a clear, colorless fluid found around the brain and spine, which makes up less than I percent of the body's water. It provides a protective buffer against shock and transports metabolic waste products, antibodies, and chemical and pathological products of disease away from the brain and spinal cord and into the bloodstream to be filtered out.

Extracellular and intracellular fluids help control the movement of water and electrolytes throughout the body. Extracellular fluid enables the absorption and excretion of water into and out of the body and supports inorganic ion exchange between the internal and external environments to maintain homeostasis.

Percutaneous Methods of Application

PRIMARY

- Neat application (of tea tree or English lavender* essential oil only, as local antiseptic/bactericidal first aid
- Compress
- Diluted in a carrier for local skin and underlying soft tissue care, whether for wound care, for skin healing, or in beauty products
- Massage oil
- Face mask/body wrap

SECONDARY

- Bath
- Perfume
- Shampoos/conditioners or hair oils
- Commercial toiletry products
- Direct contact with household and commercial cleaning products

*Spike lavender has a high camphor content, which means it is prone to be an irritant to skin unless diluted in a carrier medium.

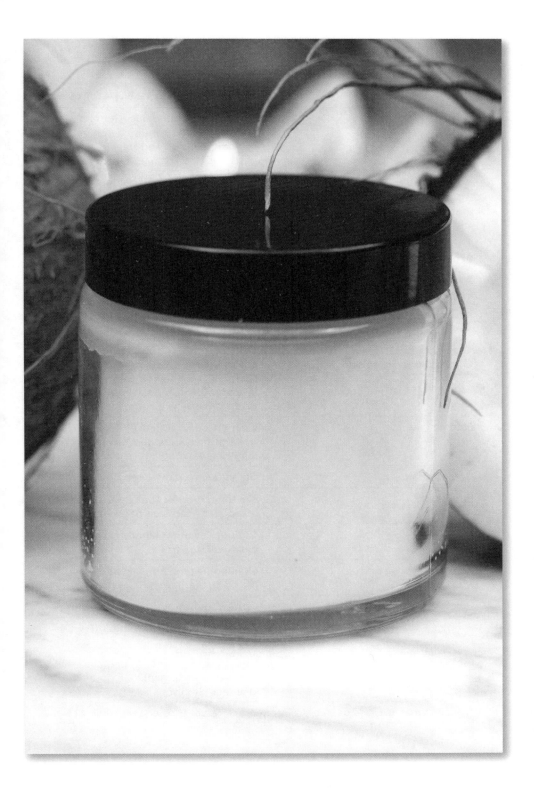

SERENITY ESSENTIAL OILS FOR
COMMON SKIN CONDITIONS

CONDITION	RECOMMENDED ESSENTIAL OILS
Abscess	Carrot seed, chamomile (German and Roman), galbanum, geranium, lavender (English and spike), patchouli, rose otto, tea tree
Acne	Cajeput, carrot seed, chamomile (German and Roman), galbanum, geranium, lavender (English and spike), mandarin, petitgrain, rose otto, tea tree, vetivert
Acne rosacea	Chamomile (German)
Bruises	Chamomile (Roman), geranium, lavender (English)
Burns*	Chamomile (German and Roman), geranium, lavender (English and spike), tea tree
Chapped or cracked skin	Cajeput, carrot seed, chamomile (German and Roman), geranium, lavender (English), patchouli, rose otto, vetivert
Eczema	Carrot seed, chamomile (Roman), frankincense, geranium, lavender (English), patchouli, rose otto
Herpes simplex	Geranium, rose otto, tea tree
Infections	See the *anti-infectious* essential oils listed in the table on page 70
Insect bites	Cajeput, lavender (English and spike), patchouli, tea tree
Itching	Chamomile (Roman), lavender (English), tea tree
Excessive perspiration	Cypress, petitgrain
Pimples	Cajeput, galbanum, lavender (English and spike), tea tree
Psoriasis	Cajeput, carrot seed, chamomile (German and Roman), galbanum, lavender (English)

*For burns that cover a large area, are infected, or affect deep tissue, seek medical help.

CONDITION	RECOMMENDED ESSENTIAL OILS
Puffiness	Chamomile (German and Roman), cypress
Ringworm	Cajeput, geranium, lavender (spike), patchouli, petitgrain, tea tree, vetivert
Scalp conditions	Dry scalp: petitgrain, rose otto; oily scalp: patchouli, petitgrain
Scars	Carrot seed, frankincense, galbanum, lavender (English), patchouli, petitgrain
Sensitive skin	Chamomile (Roman)
Shingles	Geranium, lavender (spike), tea tree

Note: Do not use essential oils neat on your skin. Instead, always dilute them in a vegetable oil or nonperfumed lotion, cream, or ointment. (The exceptions are tea tree and English lavender essential oils, which may be applied neat, or undiluted, as a first-aid treatment.)

Calendula (the essential oil and infused oil), though not a Serenity Essential Oil, is a great skin remedy. It's very effective for acne rosacea, bruises, burns, chapped or cracked skin, combination skin, eczema, itching, psoriasis, scars, and shingles.

SERENITY ESSENTIAL OILS FOR COMMON SKIN TYPES

SKIN TYPE	RECOMMENDED ESSENTIAL OIL
Combination (dry/oily) skin	Chamomile (German and Roman), cypress, frankincense, geranium, lavender (English), patchouli, rose otto
Dry skin	Carrot seed, chamomile (German and Roman), geranium (balances sebum), petitgrain (balances sebum), rose otto (balances sebum), vetivert
Mature skin	Carrot seed, cypress, frankincense, galbanum, lavender (English), patchouli, rose otto, spikenard; see also the *revitalizing* essential oils listed in the chart on the next page
Normal skin	Geranium, lavender (English), rose otto
Oily skin	Cajeput, cypress, chamomile (German), frankincense, geranium (balances sebum), lavender, mandarin, petitgrain (balances sebum), tea tree, vetivert

SERENITY ESSENTIAL OILS: MODES OF ACTION

MODES OF ACTION	ESSENTIAL OILS
Antifungal	Depends on the type of fungus; see the chart on pages 72–74
Anti-infectious	Cajeput, chamomile (German and Roman), cypress, galbanum, lavender (English and spike), patchouli, petitgrain, spikenard, tea tree
Anti-inflammatory	Carrot seed, chamomile (German), cypress, frankincense, galbanum, lavender (English and spike), patchouli, petitgrain, rose otto, tea tree
Antiseptic	Cajeput, cypress, lavender (spike), patchouli, tea tree
Astringent	Cypress, frankincense, galbanum, geranium, patchouli, rose otto
Bactericide	All Serenity Essential Oils to varying degrees, but especially cajeput, chamomile (German), cypress, geranium, lavender (English and spike), mandarin, patchouli, rose otto, and tea tree
Deodorant	Cypress, geranium, lavender (English), patchouli, petitgrain, spikenard
Hydrating	Mandarin, rose otto
Immune support	Chamomile (German and Roman), lavender (English and spike), patchouli, tea tree
Purifying	Lavender (English and spike), mandarin, tea tree
Revitalizing	Carrot seed, tea tree
Toner	Chamomile (Roman), frankincense, lavender (English), mandarin, petitgrain, rose otto

The human microbiome consists of trillions of microbes, including fungi, which live symbiotically on and in the body—on the skin, in the gut, and in cavities such as the mouth, ears, and vagina. The microbiome plays a significant role in protecting and maintaining immunity and aids a number of bodily functions: for example, assisting the breakdown and digestion of food in the gut, and providing a protective barrier against invasion from harmful microbes and pathogens. Poor diet, sugary refined foods, overuse of antibiotics, some pharmaceutical drugs, stress, and illness, among other factors, can disrupt the harmonious balance of the microbiome. There are approximately 350 known pathogenic fungi. Many, like *Candida albicans*, coexist healthily within the microbiome and only become harmful if their proliferation is unchallenged and they spread into other areas of the body.

All essential oils are antifungal, antimicrobial, and antiviral, to varying degrees. Their antifungal effects are attributed to the ability of terpene and terpinoid compounds, prevelant within all essential oils, to kill fungal cells and/or to prevent their proliferation (Nazzaro et al. 2017). Christopher Vasey, in his important work *Natural Antibiotics and Antivirals,* points out that the molecular complexity of essential oils makes it difficult for pathogens to develop resistance to them. Certain essential oils, due to their specific chemical content, will be more effective than others against invasive fungi. Vasey (2018, 110) identifies oregano, palmarosa, savory, tea tree, and thyme as broad spectrum (that is, antifungal, antiseptic, antiviral) essential oils; tea tree is the most versatile. The charts below list the most common types of invasive fungi and the essential oils most likely to be effective against them. Serenity essential oils are highlighted with boldface.

FUNGAL INFECTIONS AND PATHOGENS

AREA OF THE BODY	INFECTION	ASSOCIATED FUNGAL PATHOGENS
Hair and scalp	Tinea capitis (ringworm)	*Malassezia furfur*
		Microsporum audouinii
		Microsporum canis
		Trichophyton schoenleinii
		Trichophyton soudanense
		Trichophyton tonsurans
		Trichophyton verrucosum
		Trichophyton violaceum
Face	Tinea faciei	*Trichophyton mentagrophytes*
		Trichophyton rubrum
		Trichophyton tonsurans

FUNGAL INFECTIONS AND PATHOGENS (continued)

AREA OF THE BODY	INFECTION	ASSOCIATED FUNGAL PATHOGENS
Feet	Tinea pedis (ringworm, athlete's foot)	*Epidermophyton floccosum*
		Trichophyton mentagrophytes
		Trichophyton rubrum var. *interdigitale*
Hands	Tinea manuum	*Trichophyton mentagrophytes*
		Trichophyton rubrum
Body	Tinea corporis (ringworm, superficial fungal infections)	*Epidermophyton floccosum*
		Microsporum canis
		Trichophyton mentagrophytes
Groin	Tinea cruris (ringworm)	*Epidermophyton floccosum*
		Trichophyton rubrum
Nails	Tinea unguium (ringworm, fungal infection of nails)	*Candida* species
		Trichophyton mentagrophytes
		Trichophyton rubrum
Face and upper back	Tinea versicolor	*Malassezia furfur*

ANTIFUNGAL ESSENTIAL OILS

FUNGAL PATHOGEN	RECOMMENDED ESSENTIAL OILS (TOPICAL USE ONLY)
Candida species	Cinnamon bark *(Cinnamomum zeylanicum)**
	Fennel *(Foeniculum vulgare)*
	Geranium *(Pelargonium graveolens)*
	Lavender, English *(Lavandula angustifolia)*

*Known mucous irritant, skin irritant, and sensitizer; use in moderation; avoid during pregnancy; do not apply to babies or children; do not take internally.

See also table notes on page 74.

FUNGAL PATHOGEN	RECOMMENDED ESSENTIAL OILS (TOPICAL USE ONLY)
Candida species (continued)	Lemongrass *(Cymbopogon citratus)**
	Melissa (Lemon balm) *(Melissa officinalis)*
	Palmarosa *(Cymbopogon martinii)*
	Patchouli *(Pogostemon cablin)*
	Peppermint *(Mentha piperita)*
	Spikenard *(Nardostachys grandiflora)*
	Tea tree *(Melaleuca alternifolia)*
	Thyme *(Thymus vulgaris*—thymol and carvacrol chemotypes)*
	Vetivert *(Vetiveria zizanioides)*
Epidermophyton species	Lemongrass *(Cymbopogon citratus)**
	Spearmint *(Mentha spicata)*
	Tea tree *(Melaleuca alternifolia)*
	Vetivert *(Vetiveria zizanioides)*
Malassezia species	Cinnamon bark *(Cinnamomum zeylanicum)**
	Lavender, spike *(Lavandula latifolia)*
	Lemongrass *(Cymbopogon citratus)**
	Myrrh *(Commiphora myrrha)*
	Tea tree *(Melaleuca alternifolia)*
	Thyme *(Thymus vulgaris*—thymol and carvacrol chemotypes)*
Microsporum species	Fennel *(Foeniculum vulgare)*
	Lemon *(Citrus limon)*
	Lemongrass *(Cymbopogon citratus)**
	Spearmint *(Mentha spicata)*
	Tea tree *(Melaleuca alternifolia)*
	Thyme *(Thymus vulgaris*—thymol and carvacrol chemotypes)*
	Vetivert *(Vetiveria zizanioides)*

*Known mucous irritant, skin irritant, and sensitizer; use in moderation; avoid during pregnancy; do not apply to babies or children; do not take internally.

See also table notes on page 74.

ANTIFUNGAL ESSENTIAL OILS (continued)

FUNGAL PATHOGEN	RECOMMENDED ESSENTIAL OILS (TOPICAL USE ONLY)
Trichophyton species	Fennel *(Foeniculum vulgare)*
	Geranium *(Pelargonium graveolens)*
	Java citronella *(Cymbopogon winterianus)*
	Lavender, English *(Lavandula angustifolia)*
	Lemon *(Citrus limon)*
	Tea tree *(Melaleuca alternifolia)*
	Vetivert *(Vetiveria zizanioides)*

Note: Effective treatment of a fungal infection may require daily applications of the recommended essential oil for six to twelve months.

Dermal and nail applications: Dilute the essential oil in a water-based cream or lotion. (See chapter 7 for instructions on blending essential oils into creams and lotions.)

Love the skin you are in.

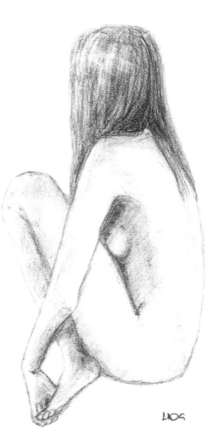

Potentially Sensitizing Essential Oils

The following essential oils may cause sensitization (a state of hyper-sensitivity). Avoid them in cases of sensitive, damaged, or diseased skin. Serenity Essential Oils are marked in bold type; use in high dilution.

Allspice	Fennel	Oregano
Aniseed	Fir needle	Orange
Basil	Ginger	Parsley
Black pepper	Juniper	Peppermint
Celery seed	Lemon	Pine
Chamomile	Lemongrass	Sage
(German and Roman)	Lime	Spearmint
Cinnamon (bark and leaf)	Marigold (*Tagetes minuta*)	**Tea tree**
Citronella	May chang (*Litsea cubeba*)	Thyme
Clary sage	Melissa	Ylang ylang
Clove (bud, leaf, and stem)	Myrtle	
Costus	Nutmeg	

Also avoid all absolutes and resinoids, which can retain chemical residue from their extraction process.

Although chamomile and tea tree are generally very gentle and nonhazardous—among the reasons they are included in the Serenity Essential Oils—they can have some potentially irritant effects for sensitive individuals. Chamomile (German and Roman) essential oil, for example, is recommended for aller-gies and sensitivities. However, due to its intense odiferous quality, it can also instigate a skin irritant reaction, so it should be applied only in moderation and at a low dose (1 percent or less dilution in a carrier medium). Tea tree, when used in high dose, especially undiluted, can cause temporary numbness or a tingling sensation to the area to which it is applied. Tea tree also causes skin to become dry, which increases propensity for irritation.

ORAL INGESTION

Essential oils are mucous membrane irritants, which means that it is unlikely that a person will "overdose" through olfaction; the irritant qualities actually act as a self-regulating mechanism. It is also unlikely that a person will "overdose" via dermal applications; the skin acts as a semiporous barrier moderating penetration by the essential oils, and the result of an excessive dosage is a rash or other skin irritation. In both cases, only a small percentage of the dose that is applied will be absorbed into the body.

In contrast, when administered orally, it is likely that 100 percent of the essential oil that is ingested will be absorbed by the body. The potential for overdose and harm is considerable. For this reason, oral ingestion of essential oils is **not** recommended unless prescribed and administered by a health-care practitioner who is also a trained and qualified essential oil practitioner. I do not advocate oral ingestion of essential oils in any other circumstance.

Essential oils should never be swallowed neat (undiluted) because they can cause severe mucous membrane irritation. Although essential oils are metabolized and excreted from the body quite quickly, there is increased risk of causing renal (kidney) and hepatic (liver) damage and internal irritation to other accessory organs of the digestive system. Some essential oils are oral toxins.

There is also increased risk of negative chemical interaction between the constituents of essential oils and other prescribed medication that may be being taken at the same time, which might potentiate or exacerbate each other's actions. For example, sweet birch or wintergreen essential oil should never be administered internally if a person is also taking warfarin, as these essential oils dangerously increase the anticoagulant and blood-thinning potential of warfarin.

In their book *Essential Oil Safety: A Guide for Health Professionals,* Tisserand and Young (2014, 58) warn of possible incompatibility between oral ingestion of the essential oils of German chamomile, chaste tree, cypress (blue), sandalwood (W. Australian), and jasmine sambac absolute and tricyclic antidepressants, such as imipramine and amitriptyline, or opiates, such as codeine, because these essential oils can potentiate the action of these drugs.

It is vital, therefore, that professional health-care practitioners, before administering or prescribing essential oils, carefully consider the following:

+ All medications and other treatments taken by or administered to their patient or client
+ The chemistry of any essential oils under consideration for administeration (to avoid adverse reactions and the potentiation of other drugs or medications, and to ensure therapeutic compatibility and appropriateness)
+ Potential contraindications that may prohibit the internal ingestion of some or all essential oils
+ The current health and physiological condition of their patient or client
+ The most appropriate route and method of administration
+ Appropriate/compatible carrying mediums (vegetable/plant oil, honey, tincture, soluble capsules, charcoal tablets, and so on)
+ The dose and frequency of administration
+ The duration of treatment
+ The patient's response to treatment (healing response, speed of recovery, quality of healing, any exacerbation of original symptoms, development of new symptoms, side effects or negative reactions such as headache, vomiting, rash, anxiety, sensitization, and so on)

When taken internally, essential oils are usually suspended, dispersed, or dissolved in an emulsifying substance such as full-fat milk, vegetable/plant oil, or honey, or they are suspended in vegetable oil in soluble capsules and swallowed with water or, if appropriate, food in order to avoid irritation and to aid assimilation. (Note that full-fat milk does not completely emulsify essential oils.) The high rate of absorption through oral ingestion means that the dose should be controlled and monitored appropriately. For example, a safe effective dose does not normally exceed 2 to 6 drops of essential oil, taken within a twenty-four-hour period. For acute conditions, essential oils are sometimes applied at higher doses, under appropriate professional medical guidance, for short periods of time. For chronic, longer-term conditions, essential oils are applied in lower doses to accommodate prolonged usage, with breaks in between to prevent sensitization; for example, a patient might take essential oils for one to two weeks, followed by a break, or abstinence, of a week, before resuming the treatment. Changing the essential oil being used over an extended period of application can also help prevent sensitization.

Dose depends on the type of essential oil being consumed; some are more toxic than others, some should not be taken internally at all, some have little toxic or adverse effect; combinations of oils can increase or decrease toxic propensity. Dose also depends on the size and constitution of the person. It is imperative that you are fully aware of the constituents, contraindications, and related safety information of a given essential oil and combinations of essential oils before consuming or applying them. For further information regarding the safe oral ingestion of essential oils in therapy, please refer to Tisserand and Young's *Essential Oil Safety: A Guide for Health Professionals,* 2nd ed. (London: Churchill Livingstone, 2014).

ESSENTIAL OIL METABOLISM AND EXCRETION

Metabolism refers to the chemical reactions within cells that transform or synthesize substances into another form. The aim of metabolism is to create and maintain a functional balanced environment in order to support homeostasis and sustain the life of the body (or organism). The process of metabolism sets off a series of enzyme-catalyzed transformative reactions (the metabolic pathway) that enable the body (organism) to grow, reproduce, maintain structure, and respond to environmental (internal and external) changes and conditions. There are two categories of metabolism:

+ **Catabolism,** a metabolic pathway whereby, through a process known as respiration, organic matter is broken down to release energy
+ **Anabolism,** a metabolic pathway whereby energy is utilized to construct cell components, such as proteins and nucleic acids

The liver is the major organ of metabolism. However, the skin, nervous system, kidneys, lungs, intestinal mucosa, blood plasma, adrenals, and placenta also participate in this process. Enzymes, which catalyze and speed up the rate of metabolic reactions, often require vitamins and minerals found in foods (and supplements) in order to enable this function.

Essential oil molecules that reach the circulatory system eventually arrive via the bloodstream at the liver, where, through the process of metabolism, their compounds are broken down into smaller units, known as metabolites, that have various biochemical effects. A single essential oil compound may create several metabolites that ultimately bear little resemblance to the original compound. Essential oil compounds are predominantly lipophilic, yet their metabolites are less so. Metabolites are either excreted almost immediately (within minutes or a few hours) or are distributed to their site of action or bound to tissue and plasma proteins and excreted later (the duration between absorption and elimination varies from constituent to constituent but does not appear to extend much beyond 72 to 120 hours) (Tisserand and Young 2014, 53–57).

The waste products of metabolism are eliminated from the body via the kidneys (urine), lungs (breath), and skin (perspiration), and, to a certain extent, within exudates from other orifices, such as feces, mucus, and earwax.

Damian and Damian (1995, 55) encapsulate the physiological and psychological pathways of essential oils in their succinct diagram (see page 80), demonstrating the extensive influence essential oils may have on the systems of the body, including the brain.

〜

Compared to percutaneous absorption, olfaction does seem to offer the most expedient route into the body. Essential oil molecules passing through the nose and olfactory epithelium initiate an immediate neurological, psycho-emotional response within the brain, affecting mood, emotion, and perception and triggering hormone release via the hypothalamus and pituitary gland.

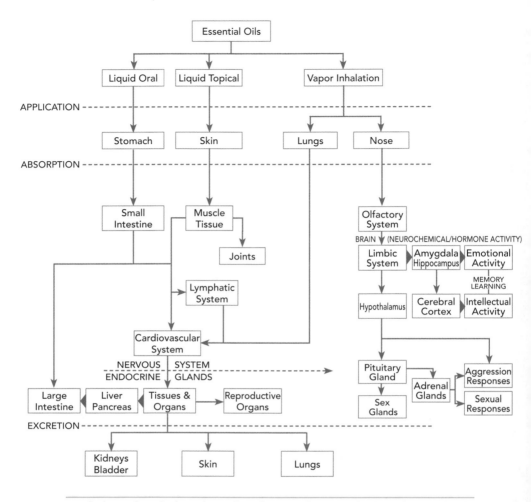

Psychological and physiological pathways of essential oils within the body (Adapted from Peter and Kate Damian's *Aromatherapy: Scent and Psyche*)

Essential oil molecules find their way into the circulatory system through diffusion into capillaries in the nose and respiratory tract but mostly via the alveoli in the lungs. Due to their skin and mucous membrane irritant effect, essential oils can be administered only in limited quantity via this route, so an "overdose" is unlikely. Only a small amount of essential oil is necessary to procure a psycho-emotional or hormonal response, so this limit does not inhibit their potential.

Percutaneous absorption, however, is impeded by the barrier effect of the skin. Essential oils are hydrophobic and naturally move with ease from water-based mediums (creams and lotions) to bind with lipids found in skin. However, diffusion through the skin (which is both lipophilic and hydrophilic) takes time (up to twenty-four hours) and occurs at varying rates according to the type of molecules comprising the essential oil and their pathway through the dermis. While molecules do eventually find their way into the bloodstream and to underlying organs, many remain suspended in the epidermis and/or evaporate from the skin. Yet, as previously mentioned in this chapter, essential oils do have a far-reaching effect when applied topically. Percutaneous absorption works very well for topical conditions such as dermatitis, wound healing, and arthritis (especially where there is inflammation), and it also initiates psycho-emotional effects (via both percutaneous absorption and incidental inhalation).

Both olfaction and percutaneous absorption appear to influence hormone release and support the immune system, which may stimulate or sedate the nervous system and, due to the antimicrobial properties of certain molecules, offer protection against and combat pathogens.

The Predominant Therapeutic Actions and Benefits of Essential Oils

- Stimulate an endocrine response: endorphin and hormone release (affecting mood, emotion, perception, attitude, nervous system, and physiological function)
- Stimulate and sedate (physiologically and psycho-emotionally)
- Calm or invigorate (physiologically and psycho-emotionally)
- Strengthen and support the immune system
- Combat infections
- Support skin healing and tissue regeneration
- Enhance, reinforce, and strengthen memory, increasing the salience of experiential memory and recall of emotions, events, and information

3

Safe Practice

Boundaries of Use and Contraindications

Used sensibly, essential oils pose little risk and provide tremendous benefit. Indeed, essential oils have become increasingly popular, particularly in the integrated health and beauty industries, and are promoted as ingredients in commercial household products and foods ranging from air fresheners and fabric conditioners to flavored coffees and exotic foodstuffs—the words *aroma* and *aromatic,* strategically placed in the language of advertisements, apparently taking full advantage of this popularity. However, the portayal of essential oils in some promotional images—as being primarily useful for pampering, relaxing, or indulging oneself—may serve to trivialize and to detract attention not only from their significant therapeutic benefit, but also from the fact that they are distilled chemical derivatives of plants and as such require sensible handling and application. It is true that relaxation and an enhanced sense of self-worth can be positive outcomes of essential oil applications. However, essential oils do possess many other qualities too (as testified to in the rest of this book)—and potential hazards as well.

The term *essential oil* is itself misleading. Essential oils alone are not emollient. They are considered "essential" in the sense that they carry a distinctive scent, or essence, of the plant (European Chemicals Agency 2019). But they are not emollient, as you would expect an oil to be. In contrast, when applied neat to the skin, they tend to be drying and are potential irritants and sensitizers.

There are numerous aromatherapy texts extolling the virtues of essential oils (including this one), citing benefits that range from antipathogenic to wound care and skin-healing properties, not to mention psycho-emotional effects and hedonistic enjoyment. While this information is valuable, it also poses a dilemma; that is, boundaries of appropriate application and practice are not always clearly identified. Tisserand and Young (2014), addressing this anomaly, provide comprehensive essential oil safety guidance in their book *Essential Oil Safety: A Guide for Health Professionals.* However, many books do not—and thus the boundary between the layperson and the professional practitioner is sometimes blurred or obscured through lack of being clearly acknowledged.

I am not suggesting that these books are not valuable and informative—indeed, many of them have informed my own journey of learning and discovery—but I do believe that overlooking or not clearly identifying the boundaries of expertise for specialized fields of health and well-being encourages preponderance toward trivialization at best, and inappropriate remedy at worst. It also panders to the critic who aims to channel all health-care options and choice toward the pharmaceutical industry and away from the individual.

Some aromatherapy texts seem to focus on remedies for ailments related to chronic stress, while others also include remedies for serious medical conditions that require professional diagnosis and support. To illustrate, one author recommends oral ingestion of *Melaleuca alternifolia* (tea tree) essential oil (1 to 3 drops every half hour with "lots of water or herbal tea") for bladder infections (Schnaubelt 1999, 103)—but bladder infections can indicate a range of underlying conditions from cystitis in women to prostate cancer in men. Another prescribes *Rosmarinus officinalis* (rosemary) essential oil for hypercholesterolemia (high cholesterol levels in the blood) and jaundice (yellowing of the eyes and skin due to poor liver function) (Lawless 1995, 209); both are serious conditions that require professional medical attention.

Directly or by implication, these authors suggest ingestion of essential oils as a treatment for some of the conditions cited (liver dysfunction, high cholesterol, bladder infection, and so on). It is not always clear whether inhalation or percutaneous absorption of the essential oils being cited would also be an effective route of administration for such conditions, and sometimes the method of application is not specified. Equally, the authors do not always clarify whether the therapeutic properties they cite for an essential oil are for the essential oil itself or for the whole plant—and we must remember that essential oils comprise only the volatile chemicals of the plant.

Essential oils added to herbal teas (as above) can possibly alter the chemical composition of the herbal infusion, which may enhance or negate any potential therapeutic action (or reaction); a sound knowledge of herbalism, anatomy, physiology, and pathology is a prerequisite before administering essential oils in this way. Only professional practitioners who are appropriately qualified and carry out a thorough consultation with their client should recommend such remedies.

As discussed in chapter 2, interactions can sometimes occur between medications (whether prescription or over the counter) and certain essential oils. In addition, some essential oils may exacerbate symptoms of dysfunction. For example, someone being treated for severe anxiety may find that some essential oils intensify or, conversely, counteract the effect of their medication, or they may mimic the symptomatic experienced feelings of anxiety (racing heart, feeling nervous/excited/fearful or overwhelmed) because these oils are too stimulating for them at that moment in time. Such symptoms can also occur when a person is experiencing a sensitized reaction to one or all of the components within a particular essential oil.

Some aromatherapy journals and books are clearly aimed at biomedical clinical practitioners, especially nurses. We find, for example, the *International Journal of Clinical Aromatherapy,* Buckle's *Clinical Aromatherapy: Essential Oils in Practice,* and Bensouilah and Buck's *Aromadermatology: Aromatherapy in the Treatment and Care of Common Skin Conditions,* among others. However, many aromatherapy texts are written for the lay reader or budding aromatherapy student.

Robert Tisserand, in his groundbreaking book *The Art of*

Aromatherapy, reminds us that essential oils are, indeed, multidynamic with capacity to influence at one and the same time physiological, psycho-emotional, and spiritual responses. The result is that essential oils can be applied in quite different ways in a variety of contexts—from beauty and massage to remedial applications. Tisserand acknowledges that the term *aromatherapy* is inclusive and also implies the ability of essential oils to simply make us feel good. As he acknowledges, the transcending sensual pleasantness of their scents can be inspiring, uplifting, and soothing, and feeling better can have a tremendous psychosomatic influence on stress-related illnesses and conditions.

Due to their multidynamic qualities, essential oils are adaptable and as such are effectively applied within a range of health-care modalities, such as nursing, midwifery, dermatology, physiotherapy, palliative care, behavioral psychology, counseling, and mindfulness meditation, and in "self-help" formulations and remedies for stress, relaxation, and well-being. They also feature in aesthetic and beauty formulations and other manufactured products. When applying essential oils in any of the above contexts, knowledge, skill, and clearly defined boundaries of practice and administration are observed in the interest of safe and effective application.

To be clear, this book aims to support those who wish to manage and enhance their personal well-being as a preventive measure. It is not intended as a substitute for other appropriate professional health care.

AROMATHERAPY IN CONTEXT: BOUNDARIES OF APPLICATION

The Complementary and Natural Healthcare Council (CNHC) in the United Kingdom describes aromatherapy as "the therapeutic use of essential oils to help deal with everyday stresses and emotional well-being." The National Center for Complementary and Integrative Health (NCCIH) in the United States describes aromatherapy as "the use of essential oils from plants (flowers, herbs, or trees) as therapy to improve physical, mental, and spiritual well-being" (2019). Tisserand and Young (2014, 2) describe aromatherapy as "the use of essential oils, applied topically, orally, by inhalation, or other means, to promote health, hygiene and psycho-logical well-being." The latter definition implies four potential and loosely overlapping modes of using and applying essential oils:

+ Medicinal
+ Psycho-emotional
+ Dermatological (skin care)
+ Environmental

Damian and Damian (1995, 12) broadly organize the use and application of essential oils into three categories:

1. **Clinical/medical,** which involves internal ingestion for systemic conditions and viral/bacterial invasion, illness, or disease, and topical application for wound care and skin conditions
2. **Aesthetic/cosmetic,** which involves topical application for beauty treatments and skin care and appearance, integrity, and rejuvenation
3. **Holistic/naturopathic,** which involves topical application and/or aromatic inhalation for hedonistic enjoyment and psycho-emotional or physiological stress-related chronic conditions, and for the general support and maintenance of health and well-being

Diagnosis of illness or disease and the subsequent prescription of medicine or medical treatment (category 1) require that the therapist has specialized clinical, biomedical, herbalist, or pharmaceutical training and is licensed to practice medicine; such licenses are typically tightly controlled by government bodies. The creation, application, and retail of cosmetic products and procedures (category 2) are generally heavily regulated. Holistic and naturopathic remedial practice and application (category 3) are also typically controlled and regulated. Thus, there are contextual boundaries of practice implicit within the above definitions of aromatherapy and consequential regulations that require consideration when applying essential oils, whether as a professional therapeutic modality or even for "self-help" wellness management.

Such laws and regulations help ensure that essential oils, and other related products, applied for personal use, are monitored and appropriately managed through the line of supply (from field to home). But it is also up to individuals to acknowledge their own limits and boundaries in terms of their application of essential oils.

A professional aromatherapist works within a holistic health-care framework, whether as a sole practitioner or as an employee of a larger organization. When applying essential oils in the context of professional practice, it is important to be clear about boundaries and responsibility for care and protection. Aromatherapists working in a clinical context (for example, in a medical clinic, hospital, hospice, nursing home, school, or other supportive setting), regardless of whether they are also a trained nurse or other health-care professional, teacher, or caregiver, must first gain consent from the clinical manager, doctor, or other specialist in charge before applying essential oils to others (whether for therapeutic, personal hygiene, or beauty purposes). They must also gain consent from the person who will be receiving the treatment (or from an adult guardian, if they are working with children).

Essential Oils and Integrity

There are two areas of responsibility to consider when applying essential oils (whether for personal or professional therapeutic use):

Essential oil integrity: appropriate, sustainable growing, harvesting, and extraction methods; authenticity and purity; appropriate storage, handling, use, and application; evidence of appropriate certification (laboratory evaluation, safety data, and other quality control information)

User integrity: adherence to appropriate professional boundaries of application, practice, and context; appropriate knowledge and awareness of the nature of essential oils and pathophysiological diagnosis (ability to identify which conditions or symptoms require referral to an appropriate health-care professional, which are suitable for professional collaborative treatment, and which are symptoms of stress and/ or are stress related and would benefit from aromatherapeutic treatment); appropriate application and well-being management

---

The essential oil and aromatherapy industry is regulated. Essential oil suppliers are obliged to provide safety data information to the consumer. As the end user, the consumer is permitted to apply the products of this industry for personal use. However, if a person wants to apply, redistribute, or sell these products to others, then he or she also must adhere to the established safety regulations and protocols. Appropriate professional training is a significant aspect of safety protocol when applying essential oils to others, alongside ensuring that essential oils are sourced from appropriately regulated, reputable suppliers.

Aromatherapy Training

Professional aromatherapy training is generally broken into two categories to accommodate the context of practice:

+ **Essential Oil Practitioner (EOP):** applies essential oils in the form of massage and other topical applications via skin-care products such as lotions, creams, gels, ointments, clays, and compresses, as well as by steam inhalations, therapeutic perfumes, and so on.
+ **Essential Oil Therapist or Technician (EOT):** applies essential oils in all of the above ways but omits massage as a delivery vehicle and places greater focus on preparing remedies for clients' self-application using nasal inhalers, personal therapeutic perfumes, vaporization (environmental diffusers, steam inhalation), and skin-care products.

The underpinning training remains the same for both routes. Professional aromatherapists then will focus on a particular client group (e.g., palliative and elderly care, managing stress in the workplace, beauty and well-being, and so on), apply their skills in conjunction with other health and well-being skills (training as a nurse, physiotherapist, herbalist, acupuncturist, counselor, beautician, and so on), or set up practice as an independent therapist treating stress or stress-related conditions to aid well-being. Each country will have its own professional training schools and awarding bodies. A weekend course is great as an introduction, but adequate and appropriate aromatherapy training will take time (a year or more).

Whatever their purview, aromatherapists work (directly or indirectly) with other health-care professionals and must adhere to contextual and appropriate protocols, limitations, and professional boundaries. For example, professional aromatherapists can treat stress and the symptoms of stress, but a stress-related condition must be diagnosed by their client's primary-care physician (or other appropriate health-care professional) to eliminate all other potential systemic or pathogenic causes. The same principle applies to individuals using essential oils for personal self-help.

Aromatherapists are not licensed to diagnose or prescribe essential oils as medicine unless they are professionally trained to do so; if they do observe symptoms that may indicate an underlying medical condition, disease, or illness, they must advise their client to seek appropriate professional diagnosis from their primary-care physician or other appropriate medical practitioner.

Boundaries are a safeguarding mechanism. Professional specialized skills and expertise are honed and developed inside these boundaries. For example, aromatherapists can (valuably) apply counseling skills to the therapeutic interaction with their client, but this does not give them license to take on the role of a psychotherapist (in spite of their good intention), which would require additional specialized training, qualification, and, significantly, professional supervision; once professionally trained, aromatherapists may then apply both modalities as complements to each other. Conversely, professional health-care practitioners must ensure that they are adequately trained, qualified, and knowledgeable about essential oils before applying or prescribing them to their clients or patients.

The consultation process enables aromatherapists (or any health-care professional) the opportunity to determine whether aromatherapy will benefit their client; in this context, both therapist and client collaborate and each has a responsibility to clearly communicate and identify limitations and boundaries and provide sufficient relevant information to enable implementation of an appropriate treatment plan. In lieu of this process, when using essential oils for self-help health and wellness maintenance, although it may seem pedantic, the user is advised to first consider a quick self-consultation or "check-in" process, as outlined below.

Self-Consultation: Preparation for Self-Treatment

INITIAL ASSESSMENT

Primary condition or reason for seeking treatment: _____

_____

Secondary conditions or reasons for seeking treatment (if applicable):

_____

Desired outcome of treatment: _____

TREATMENT PLAN

Appropriate method of application: _____

Appropriate essential oil(s): _____

Appropriate carrier mediums: _____

Duration and frequency of application or use: _____

_____

Potential contraindications or cautions in relation to the chosen essential oils

or carrier mediums: _____

CURRENT HEALTH STATUS

Allergies or sensitivities to foods, cosmetic products, medications, or

other substances (pet fur, metals, etc.): _____

_____

Stressors (e.g., environmental, work, family, relationships, health related,

etc.): _____

Prescribed or over-the-counter medication currently being taken: _____

_____

Dietary supplements, vitamins, and minerals currently being taken: ___

_____

Other remedial treatments in use (e.g., physiotherapy, homeopathy,

acupuncture, chiropractic, osteopathy, etc.): _____

_____

Menstrual phase/pregnancy/menopausal status (if applicable): _____

_____

Reasons for Using Essential Oil(s)

ENVIRONMENTAL

- ☐ Create a pleasant themed ambience (floral, woody, fruity, citrus, herbaceous, spicy, Christmassy, summery, refreshing, sensual, and so on)
- ☐ Use as perfume (attractant, sensual, mood-enhancing, signature or personal expression)
- ☐ Eliminate/mask unpleasant odors

PSYCHO-EMOTIONAL

- ☐ Counteract negative feelings (depression, anxiety, grief, stress, and so on)
- ☐ Improve general mood (uplift, stimulate, invigorate, calm, relax, sedate)
- ☐ Improve memory and aid learning, concentration, focus, and mental clarity

PHYSIOLOGICAL

- ☐ Combat pathogens (bacteria, viruses, fungi), whether airborne or on/in the body
- ☐ Combat uncomfortable skin conditions (eczema, psoriasis, dermatitis, itchiness, dry skin, oily skin, etc.)
- ☐ Promote healing of wounds, rashes, and other damage to the skin
- ☐ Encourage healthy skin (revitalization and regeneration of tissue)
- ☐ Mitigate stress-related conditions, including mild infections, headaches, pain and inflammation, colds, and flu
- ☐ Ease premenstrual tension and menopausal symptoms
- ☐ Mask or deodorize body odors; cleanse.

Self-treatment is not always appropriate, and there are circumstances where professional medical advice and support is absolutely necessary. If you observe or experience any of the "red flag" symptoms or conditions listed in the box on the following page, you are advised to seek medical attention immediately.

Red Flags: Conditions That Require Immediate Medical Attention

- Blue lips
- Fever/excessive sweating
- Persistent cough and/or sore throat
- Skin rashes
- Suppurating wounds, wounds that do not heal, or inflammation extending beyond the wound site
- Unexplained shortness of breath
- Unexplained tingling or numbness
- Unexplained tissue lumps or swelling (i.e., not due to injury)
- Abdominal distension
- Changing appearance and/or size of moles
- Persistent dyspepsia
- Prolonged, persistent headaches
- Rapid weight loss
- Rectal bleeding
- Unexplained prolonged bouts of diarrhea or constipation (not caused by diet)
- Vaginal bleeding between periods, after menopause, or after sexual intercourse
- Any unexplained persistent pain
- Disorientation
- Persistently dry, itchy skin
- Persistent fatigue and/or feelings of weakness
- Persistent memory loss
- Persistent unexplained feelings of anxiety or depression, insomnia, or suicidal thoughts
- Slurred speech

GUIDELINES FOR THE SAFE USE OF ESSENTIAL OILS

Safe Application

I do not advocate the internal use of essential oils unless they are prescribed by a professional practitioner with biomedical, pharmaceutical, or herbalist training. Awareness of the chemical interactions and physiological effects of essential oils is imperative. Essential oils are highly concentrated, volatile, odiferous chemicals, with the propensity to cause irritation and sensitization and, for some people, although relatively rare, allergic reaction if not applied appropriately.

Purchasing Essential Oil

First, ensure that you purchase essential oils from a reputable supplier whose oils are fresh, correctly packaged, and appropriately labeled, and who can vouch for the integrity of the oils they supply (details of the source, location of growth, botanical family, Latin name, batch number, safety data information, and so on). Where possible, source essential oils from locally grown and distilled crops (this ensures freshness, among other reasons). Oils that are much cheaper than average are potentially not genuine and are often adulterated or bulked out with inferior, less expensive chemicals (equally, very expensive essential oils are often adulterated with cheaper substitute chemicals or essential oils to increase profit margins). Read the labels carefully to ensure that bottles or products contain 100 percent pure essential oils.

Also, only purchase essential oils stored in amber or blue glass bottles (to protect against UV light damage) with a dropper cap (this ensures careful measurement, inhibits rapid oxidization, prevents spillage, and limits accidental ingestion by children; ask for child-proof lids if necessary). Never purchase or use essential oils that have been stored in plastic bottles, and do not purchase essential oils that have been stored on brightly lit, warm shelves (these conditions degrade essential oils). Essential oils are highly flammable so should be kept away from fire (candles, et cetera) and sources of intense heat.

Second, ensure that you know the chemical and therapeutic properties and applicable contraindications and cautions in relation to the essential oil you intend to apply before you apply it.

Using Essential Oils Safely

Chapter 7 will explain the various methods of application. When applied appropriately, essential oils pose little risk. However, while their therapeutic qualities are undoubtedly highly beneficial, they are best used in limited, controlled amounts, especially when they are applied on a frequent or daily basis. As a general rule, 6 drops of essential oil per day is the appropriate safe limit for percutaneous (creams, lotions, massage oils) and direct olfactory absorption (steam inhalation, nasal inhalers). For topical use only, this dose can be temporarily higher (for example, up to 10 drops within a twenty-four-hour period) when applied short-term for acute conditions, such as combatting the flu or a mild infection. I have observed through experience that even when applied in very small amounts, essential oils can produce a very effective response.

General Cautions for Using Essential Oils

- Do not apply essential oils neat (undiluted) on the skin; instead, always dilute them in a vegetable/plant oil or nonperfumed lotion or cream. Undiluted dermal application of essential oils can lead to irritation and sensitization. Lavender and tea tree essential oils are the exception to this rule (they are often used neat as a first-aid remedy for insect stings, minor burns or skin abrasions, or mild skin infections), but even so, repeated long-term topical application of these oils is not advisable due to the risk of sensitization.

- Do not take essential oils internally.

- Keep essential oils out of the reach of children (suppliers will provide child-proof lids if requested) and away from pets.

- Accidental ingestion: *Do not induce vomiting.* Instead, drink full-fat milk, which will act as an emollient and help protect the lining of the stomach. Seek medical advice immediately. Have ready the bottle that the essential oil was stored in for identification (the label should have the botanical Latin name, batch number, sell-by date, et cetera, and the bottle will have traces of the oil if a sample is needed).

- Accidental contact with eyes: Always wash your hands after handling essential oils to avoid transferring them from your fingers to your eyes. But if you should accidentally get undiluted essential oil in your eyes, immediately flush them with vegetable/plant oil or full-fat milk, then rinse thoroughly with warm water. Sometimes diluted essential oils enter the eyes during steam inhalation, bathing, or showering; if this happens, immediately flush your eyes with warm water. In either case, if irritation or stinging persists after you have flushed your eyes, seek immediate medical attention.

- Skin reaction: If your skin becomes irritated after application of an essential oil, apply vegetable/plant oil to the area to dilute the essential oil on your skin, then thoroughly wash the area with nonperfumed soap (liquid soap, if possible) and rinse with warm water to remove any trace of the soap and essential oil. Dry the area thoroughly and apply a nonperfumed base cream (vegetable/plant oil or even butter will work if nothing else is available) to soothe the irritation, if appropriate.

- Purchase essential oils only from reputable suppliers (who will provide safety data information).

- Purchase only essential oils that are stored in amber or dark blue glass bottles with "dropper top" lids (to ensure careful measurement and prevent spillage or accidental ingestion).

- Check the sell-by date before using an essential oil, and make a note of the date on which you open a bottle. Essential oils oxidize rapidly when exposed to oxygen in the atmosphere and therefore have a limited shelf life: two years if unopened, and one year once opened (though for citrus oils, such as mandarin, the shelf life is just six months once the bottle is opened).

- Never "top up" a bottle of essential oil with more essential oil once you have opened it.

- Discard small amounts of essential oil left in a bottle or container, unless you have been rapidly using up the essential oil from the moment that you first opened the bottle.

- Replace lids immediately after use (to slow down oxidization).

- Store in a cool, dark place, away from sources of heat and direct sunlight (preferably a fridge—although some oils, such as rose otto, will solidify when very cold, they will return to a liquid state at room temperature).

- Wipe up spillages immediately (essential oils will dissolve/damage polystyrene, plastic, varnish, paint, and polished and laminated surfaces).

Patch Testing

Patch testing is a precautionary measure to ensure the safe application of an essential oil. It is not necessary and would be impractical to carry out a patch test every time an essential oil was considered for use. However, there are indicators that can guide this decision. For example, a patch test is advisable where there is:

+ A history of sensitivity or allergy to perfumes, skin-care, or household products, metals or chemicals, and so on
+ A preexisting condition such as eczema, asthma, dermatitis, or hay fever
+ Sensitivity or allergy to the particular plant that the essential oil was extracted from, as it is likely that the essential oil will trigger a similar reaction
+ Sensitivity or allergy to particular foods or processed food additives (e.g., nuts, seeds, citrus fruits, herbs, artificial flavoring, coloring, or preservatives)
+ Current or recent longterm chronic illness (which may have weakened the immune system)

Patch Test Guidelines

1. Dilute 1 to 2 drops of essential oil, or a blend of essential oils, in 0.5 to 1 ml of a carrier medium (vegetable/plant oil, cream, lotion, ointment, et cetera). Note: this is a stronger dilution than normal, applied to a very small area of skin, to ensure a reliable result.
2. Wash and dry the area of skin selected for the patch test (for example, the fold of the arm at the elbow, the wrist, or the upper forearm).
3. Apply the diluted essential oil to the test area using a cotton bud or swab.
4. Cover the test area with a nonallergenic plaster.
5. Leave in place for one to two days. Avoid contact of the patch test with water for the duration of the test.
6. Remove the plaster and observe the test area for signs of irritation.

If the patch test yields no reaction or only mild redness (1 or 2 on the ICDRG patch test scale below), you may use the essential oil as intended.

If the patch test outcome is positive (3 to 5 on the ICDRG scale), do not use that essential oil. Or, if you used a blend of essential oils, test each one separately to identify which one was the antagonist, and then adjust the blend accordingly.

International Contact Dermatitis Research Group (ICDRG) Patch Test Scale

1. No reaction.
2. Doubtful reaction: mild redness.
3. Weak positive reaction: red and slightly thickened skin.
4. Strong positive reaction: red swollen skin with individual small watery blisters.
5. Extreme positive reaction: intense redness and swelling with coalesced large blisters or spreading reaction (extending beyond the area of application).

Note: Sometimes the patch test covering causes mild redness of the skin. This type of irritant reaction should improve quickly once the patch is removed.

Measuring Essential Oils

It is important to measure essential oils carefully, as they are prone to cause skin and mucous membrane irritation and sensitivity if they are overused or inappropriately applied. Measurement percentages can seem quite complicated, especially considering that dropper-top sizes vary, rendering absolute accuracy impossible. However, in the interest of safety, essential oil quantities do need to be monitored. Therefore, as a rule of thumb, assume the averages set out in the measurement guidelines on pages 98–99.

Risk of sensitivity or irritation reactions increases when large amounts of essential oil are applied to very small areas of skin. Applying 6 drops of essential oil in a carrier medium to the whole body through massage will have negligible irritant effect, yet the same quantity of essential oil applied to a small area of skin can be irritant, particularly in sensitive areas such as the face, underarms, and so on.

Use no more than 1 or 2 drops of essential oil in a carrier medium on localized areas of skin. Keep this in mind when making first-aid ointments or face creams or lotions. When making face creams or lotions for regular use, reduce the amount of essential oils included, change the essential oil selection from time to time, and have "no essential oil" breaks occasionally.

Measurement Guide

5 ml = 100 drops of essential oil

10 ml = 200 drops of essential oil

The maximum amount of essential oil per day for a healthy adult is 6 to 10 drops. Apply for two to three weeks, followed by one week's abstinence, and repeat. Change the essential oil selection regularly.

Proportions of Essential Oil and Carrier Medium for Blend Percentages

1 drop of essential oil in 5 ml of carrier medium = 1% blend

2½ drops of essential oil in 5 ml of carrier medium = 2.5% blend

5 drops of essential oil in 5 ml of carrier medium = 5% blend

---

Appropriate Quantities

The appropriate quantities of essential oils are indicated by the age, weight, and robustness or frailty of the individual, along with other factors such as allergies or asthma. The following are the recommended number of drops and resulting blend percentages for normal adult use and for both reduced and exceptional amounts.

Reduced Amounts

I personally do not advocate direct application of essential oils for infants under twelve months, even in dilution; the superficial layers of the skin are thinner, allowing easier permeability, and internal organs are not fully matured until after this period. Infants are more inclined to develop eczema and are more prone to environmental irritants, which can include contact with essential oils. The following information is included in the interest of safety. Do not directly apply essential oils, under any circumstances, to infants between birth and three months old. For infants between three months and twenty-four months old, use the maximum dilution—that is, 1 drop of essential oil in 20 ml or more of carrier medium—and do not use herbaceous, spicy, or citrus oil.

The following amounts are appropriate for children, for those who are frail or very elderly, and for those with sensitivities, allergies, eczema, or asthma, as well as for facial blends.

(a) 1 drop of essential oil in 5 ml of carrier medium = 1% blend
2 drops of essential oil in 10 ml of carrier medium = 1% blend

(b) 1 drop of essential oil in 10 ml of carrier medium = 0.5% blend
2 drops of essential oil in 20 ml of carrier medium = 0.5% blend

(c) 1 drop of essential oil in 20 ml of carrier medium = 0.25% blend

Normal Amounts

For general and adult use:

2½ drops of essential oil in 5 ml of carrier medium = 2.5% blend
5 drops of essential oil in 10 ml of carrier medium = 2.5% blend

Acute/Exceptional Amounts

For acute, short-term occasional use. Avoid or reduce the use of known irritant oils.

5 drops of essential oil in 5 ml of carrier medium = 5% blend
10 drops of essential oil in 10 ml carrier medium = 5% blend

POTENTIAL REACTIONS
AND CONTRAINDICATIONS

The following information covers a wide range of potential negative reactions to essential oils, contraindications for their use, health conditions that warrant special precautions, and more. Where contraindicated essential oils are listed, Serenity Essential Oils are in boldface.

It is useful to keep a log of any adverse event, small or large. You will find an example of an Adverse Reaction Report in the appendix to apply as a guide. This information should be stored in a database for reference—at the very least, your own, and/or ideally one organized by a related professional body.

Essential Oils to Avoid in Aromatherapy

These essential oils contain toxic components and should not be included in aromatherapy preparations or products (Tisserand and Balacs 1995, 339). While they are rarely sold over the counter or via mail order for public use, these essential oils do appear in pharmaceutical and other commercial formulations and so may be available through other purchasing routes.

Armoise (common or white wormwood) *(Artemisia vulgaris, A. herba-alba)*

Basil (high estragole chemotype) *(Ocimum basilicum, O. gratissimum, O. tenuiflorum)*

Bitter almond (unrectified) *(Prunus dulcis var. amara)*

Black tea tree *(Melaleuca bracteata)*

Boldo *(Peumus boldus)*

Buchu *(Agathosma crenulata)*

Cade juniper (unrectified) *(Juniperus oxycedrus)*

Calamus (triploid form—European or sweet flag) *(Acorus calamus)*

Camphor (brown or yellow) *(Cinnamomum camphora)*

Cassia (Chinese cinnamon) *(Cinnamomum cassia)*

Cinnamon bark (true cinnamon) *(Cinnamomum verum)*

Costus *(Saussurea costus)*

Elecampane *(Inula helenium)*

Fig leaf *(Ficus carica)*

Horseradish *(Armoracia rusticana)*

Lanyana (African wormwood) *(Artemisia afra)*

Mugwort (common or great) *(Artemisia vulgaris A. herba-alba, A. arborescens)*

Mustard (seeds) *(Brassica nigra, B. juncea)*

Pennyroyal *(Hedeoma pulegioides, Mentha pulegium)*

Ravensara (bark) *(Ravensara anisata)*

Sage (Dalmatian) *(Salvia officinalis)* (Spanish) *(S. lavandulifolia)*

Sassafras (Brazilian) *(Nectandra sanguinea)* (Chinese) *(Cinnamomum porrectum)*

Snakeroot (wild ginger) *(Asarum canadense)*

Sweet birch *(Betula lenta)*

Tansy *(Tanacetum vulgare)*

Tarragon *(Artemisia dracunculus)*

Tea *(Camellia sinensis)*

Thuja (northern white cedar) *(Thuja occidentalis)*

Verbena (lemon and white) *(Aloysia triphylla)*

Wintergreen *(Gaultheria fragrantissima, G. procumbens)*

Wormseed *(Chenopodium ambrosioides)*

Wormwood (high thujone content) *(Artemisia absinthium)*

Skin Reactions to Essential Oils

Essential oils tend to be drying and potentially irritant to the skin and mucous membranes, particularly when applied neat, because they are highly concentrated chemical derivatives. Skin reactions vary considerably from one individual to another, are difficult to predict, and tend to be dose dependent—that is, the concentration and quantity applied are contributory factors. Undiluted essential oils applied to damaged, diseased, or inflamed skin greatly increase the risk of a negative dermal reaction, may potentially worsen the original condition, and also significantly increase the risk of sensitization. Other factors that may influence the propensity for reactions include:

✦ Location of application or exposure

✦ Total area of skin exposed

✦ Frequency and duration of exposure

✦ Essential oil used

✦ Carrier medium used

✦ Age of recipient (children and people over the age of fifty-six are more susceptible to irritation)

✦ Pregnancy or menopause (the fluctuation of hormones in pregnant and menopausal women tends to make them hypersensitive to certain chemicals, and women's skin becomes thinner and dryer with the onset of menopause)

✦ Environment (seasonal conditions, humidity, ambient room temperature, et cetera)

✦ Whether the site of application is occluded (covered)

✦ Whether the recipient has preexisting sensitivities or allergies

✦ Whether the recipient is taking medication or using skin-care products or perfumes that may negatively interact with certain essential oils

As a precaution, people who present with allergies (nuts, dust mites, pollen, et cetera), food sensitivities, eczema, asthma, or hay fever are advised to undergo a patch test (see page 96) before using an essential oil. Also, anyone taking medication is advised to check with their prescribing physician or pharmacist before applying an essential oil to ensure that there are no known contraindications or potential for undesirable drug interaction. Safety data sheets identifying known hazards and risks (toxicity, adverse reactions, effects of overexposure, and so on) are obtainable from reputable essential oil suppliers.

The three main forms of skin reaction to essential oils are:

✦ Irritation

✦ Sensitization

✦ Phototoxicity

Irritation

Irritation manifests as redness, itchiness, burning, or stinging of the skin or mucous membranes, with or without accompanying inflammation. Skin reactions are generally classified as follows (Bensouilah and Buck 2006, 40):

✦ **Acute irritation:** local, reversible, temporary, nonimmunological inflammatory and/or noninflammatory response (redness and/or itching, burning, stinging).

+ **Irritant contact dermatitis:** acute toxic insult—for example, through exposure to acids or alkalis—and cumulative damage from repeated use of irritants.

+ **Corrosion:** irreversible, permanent alteration and disintegration of tissue at the location of contact (may manifest as inflammation, burns, and blistering). Skin is repaired with scar tissue.

The respiratory tract is particularly susceptible to irritation from essential oils. Some essential oils that are useful as inhalants for conditions affecting the respiratory system (sore throat, bronchitis, et cetera) should be applied only in low doses and for a short duration to avoid respiratory irritation. Phenols and aromatic aldehydes tend to be the most irritant essential oil compounds. Examples include eugenol (found in basil, cinnamon bark, and clove), thymol (in basil and thyme), carvacrol (in thyme, oregano, and savory), and cinnamic aldehyde (in cinnamon leaf).

Absolutes are inclined to cause irritation due to the presence of solvent chemicals in their mixture.

Essential Oils That May Cause Irritation

Basil *(Ocimum basilicum)*

Black pepper *(Piper nigrum)*

Cinnamon (bark, leaf) *(Cinnamomum verum)*

Clove (bud, leaf, stem) *(Syzgium aromaticum)*

Fennel *(Foeniculum vulgare)*

Ginger *(Zingiber officinale)*

Juniper *(Juniperus communis)*

Peppermint *(Mentha × piperita)*

Rosemary *(Rosmarinus officinalis)*

Thyme *(Thymus vulgaris)*

Verbena (lemon and white) *(Aloysia triphylla)*

Essential Oils That May Cause Irritation in People with Known Sensitivities*

Basil (high estragole chemotype) *(Ocimum basilicum, O. gratissimum, O. tenuiflorum)*

Clary sage *(Salvia sclarea)*

Geranium *(Pelargonium × asperum)*

Ginger *(Zingiber officinale)*

Grapefruit *(Citrus × paradisi)*

Gully gum *(Eucalyptus smithii)*

Lemon *(Citrus limon)*

Niaouli *(Melaleuca quinquernervia)*

Orange *(Citrus sinensis, C. × aurantium)*

Scotch pine *(Pinus sylvestris)*

Spikenard *(Nardostachys grandiflora)*

Tea tree *(Melaleuca alternifolia)*

Ylang ylang *(Cananga odorata)*

*These sensitivities include hyperreactive conditions like eczema, asthma, food allergies, and so on, which may indicate that a person is predisposed to having a negative reaction to essential oils.

Sensitization

Sensitization is not the same as sensitive skin. Sensitization is a contact hypersensitive or allergic reaction and/or severe irritation that involves the immune system (T lymphocytes and macrophages). T-lymphocyte cells become sensitized through an adaptive, exaggerated, or inappropriate immune response; once sensitized, even a small amount of the agonist substance can cause a reaction. Macrophages regulate lymphocyte activation and proliferation. Sensitization is *not* dose dependent and is difficult to predict.

The saturation point of chemical exposure can be reached through contact with products other than essential oils, such as cosmetics, perfumes, household cleaning materials, and so on. There can also be an insidious cumulative effect, especially when the same products are used repeatedly. Symptoms of sensitization are various and may include skin irritation, rashes, headaches, migraine, anxiety, heart palpitations, feelings of unease, shortness of breath, and dry mouth.

All essential oils are potential sensitizers and therefore should be applied in moderation, with regular breaks or abstinence from use (two to three weeks of use followed by a week of abstinence), and periodic rotation of the essential oils applied (substituting one oil for another, as appropriate), especially if the essential oils are being used regularly over a long period of time.

Essential Oils with Greater Propensity for Sensitization

Citrus (any kind)*

Cade juniper (unrectified) *(Juniperus oxycedrus)*

Cinnamon (bark, leaf) *(Cinnamomum verum)*

Lemongrass (East Indian) *(Cymbopogon flexuosus, C. citratus)*

May chang *(Litsea cubeba)*

Pine (any kind)* *(Pinus sylvestris, P. strobus, P. resinosa,*
    P. ponderosa, P. mugo, P. nigra)

Tea tree *(Melaleuca alternifolia)*

---

*Citrus and pine essential oils oxidize readily (a process that eventually degrades the essential oil), and oxidized essential oils are prone to causing sensitization.

Toxicity

Toxicity refers to the strength of a poison. A toxic substance damages or destroys an organism, whether the whole organism, such as a plant or animal, or a substructure of the organism, such as a cell or organ, such as the liver (hepatotoxicity) or kidney (nephrotoxicity). Damage may be reversible or irreversible, depending on the level of biological disruption and whether the regenerative capacity of the affected cells has been compromised.

Toxicity is dose dependent and is influenced by factors such as the route of administration (skin absorption, ingestion, inhalation), duration of exposure, frequency of exposure, the genetic makeup of the individual, and the individual's general state of health. Localized toxicity usually affects the organs of elimination (stomach, liver, kidneys, intestines, lungs, and skin). A toxic reaction instigated by essential oil molecules can manifest at the point of topical application or systemically.

Some essential oil molecules that may otherwise be nontoxic can bind with compounds contained in medications (most of which are toxic substances) or certain foods, or with certain enzymes, and be metabolized into a toxic substance. Chemical components within essential oils can also become toxic when they oxidize and degrade. Old essential oils are more likely to be toxic than freshly extracted, appropriately stored essential oils; this is especially true for citrus and pine essential oils.

Camphor, methyl salicylate compounds, and clove, cinnamon, and eucalyptus essential oils are most frequently cited as causes of systemic toxicity in humans. Essential oils containing phenols, fragrant aldehydes, and oxidized terpenes are the main culprits for causing dermal toxicity and irritation.

Most reported essential oil poisoning incidents involve children under six years old who accidently ingest the oils.

Phototoxicity

Phototoxicity is an excessive reaction to sunlight (or UV light, including UV light emissions from sun-tanning lamps) induced by certain chemicals present within the superficial layers of the skin. Phototoxic substances (such as the furanocoumarins found in a few essential oils, including bergamot and angelica root) absorb UV light, which in turn causes the production of abnormally dark pigmentation (brown patches), which may last for years, and reddening and burning of the surrounding skin, which is often slow to heal. A phototoxic reaction occurs only if the sensitizing agent is present. Avoid using phototoxic essential oils on skin that will be exposed to sunlight, UV light, or sun-tanning lamps. If you have applied a phototoxic essential oil, wait at least twelve to eighteen hours before exposing your skin to sunlight, UV light, or sun-tanning lamps.

Phototoxic Essential Oils

STRONG PHOTOTOXICITY

Angelica root *(Angelica archangelica)*

Bergamot (expressed unrectified) *(Citrus bergamia)*

Cumin *(Cuminum cyminum)*

Lime (expressed) *(Citrus × aurantifolia)*

Opopanax *(Commiphora guidottii)*

Rue *(Ruta graveolens)*

Marigold *(Tagetes minuta)*

Verbena absolute *(Aloysia triphylla, Lippia alba)*

MODERATE PHOTOTOXICITY

Grapefruit (expressed) *(Citrus × paradisi)*

Lemon (expressed) *(Citrus × limon)*

Orange (expressed) *(Citrus × aurantium, C. sinensis)*

Note: Please refer to Tisserand and Young's *Essential Oil Safety,* 2nd edition, for more information about the irritant potential, sensitization, and toxicity of essential oils and their chemical components.

Allergic Reactions

An allergy is a hypersensitive reaction (triggered by overstimulation of the immune system) to certain foreign substances, known as allergens. Almost anything can become an allergen; common examples include specific foods (nuts, eggs, soy, shellfish, and so on), dust mites, pollen, pet dander, and certain drugs or chemicals. Upon exposure to an allergen, immunoglobulin (an antibody produced by blood plasma) over-activates the production of white blood cells, causing an inflammatory response that can range from uncomfortable (itchiness, rashes) to dangerous (anaphylactic shock).

Anaphylaxis requires immediate medical attention; at worst it can be fatal. Its onset can be rapid, with symptoms manifesting over minutes or hours. Symptoms include throat swelling, low blood pressure, and an itchy rash. Other, less extreme allergic symptoms may include itchiness, swelling, or blistering of the skin or red, itchy, watery eyes, as well as runny nose, sneezing, rash, hives, or an asthma attack.

Obviously, people with nut allergies or sensitivities should avoid nut oils (almond, walnut, hazelnut, macadamia, coconut) as carrier mediums, and they should also avoid oils extracted from kernels (peach, apricot), which have the potential to trigger cross-reactivity. Those with wheat allergies should avoid wheat germ oil.

Potential Chemical Allergens in Essential Oils

Benzyl alcohol (ylang ylang)

Benzyl benzoate (ylang ylang, cinnamon)

Benzyl cinnamate (benzoin)

Benzyl salicylate (ylang ylang)

Cinnamic aldehyde (cinnamon)

Citral (may chang, melissa)

Citronellol (citronella)

Eugenol (cinnamon, basil)

Farnesol (rose otto)

Geraniol (geranium, palmarosa)

Limonene/D-limonene (citrus, pine, mint)

Linalool (rosewood, English lavender, camphor)

Note: The essential oils listed with these chemical compounds are only examples; there are many more essential oils that contain these compounds.

Epilepsy

Epileptic seizures are the result of excessive and abnormal cortical nerve cell activity in the brain. The systemic cause of epilepsy is generally unknown. It may develop after brain injury, a stroke, brain cancer, or drug and alcohol abuse. Reflex epilepsy caused by exposure to a certain scent is very uncommon; cases that have been reported involved mainly nonepileptics. Most reported cases of seizures induced by essential oils involve oral ingestion and mainly involve nonepileptics (Tisserand and

Young 2014, 131–39). Some essential oils, however, do contain compounds with a potential convulsive potency and should be avoided by people with known epilepsy, children, the very elderly, and pregnant women, and they should be used with caution and in low dilution in all other circumstances.

Essential Oils That Are Potentially Convulsive

Balsamite (camphor chemotype) *(Chrysanthemum balsamita)*

Camphor (yellow) (high safrol type) *(Cinnamomum camphora)*

Ho leaf (camphor/safrole chemotype) *(Cinnamomum camphora)*

Hyssop *(Hyssopus officinalis)*

Lavender (spike) *(Lavandula latifolia)*

Lavender cotton *(Santolina chamaecyparissus)*

Mugwort (common or great) *(Artemisia vulgaris, A. herba-alba, A. arborescens)*

Pennyroyal *(Hedeoma pulegioides, Mentha pulegium)*

Rosemary *(Rosmarinus officinalis)*

Sage (wild mountain) (high farnescene) *(Hemizygia petiolata)*

Tansy *(Tanacetum vulgare)*

Thuja *(Thuja occidentalis, T. plicata)*

Wormwood *(Artemisia absinthium)*

Yarrow *(Achillea millefoleum, A. nobilis)*

Cancer

Essential oils should not be used during chemotherapy or radiotherapy treatment periods. Post-treatment, essential oils must be used only in collaboration with the patient's primary health-care practitioner. Tisserand (2015) recommends avoiding essential oils for one week before chemotherapy or radiation, during treatment, and for one month afterward, hypothesizing that because many essential oils have protective antioxidant effects on our cells, there is a reasonable chance that they will do the same for cancer cells—that is, protect them from chemotherapy.

Essential Oils to Avoid in Cases of Cancer

GENERAL

Basil (estrangole CT) *(Ocimum basilicum)* (Madagascan) *(O. gratissimum)*

Fennel (bitter and sweet) *(Foeniculum vulgare)*

Ho leaf *(Cinnamomum camphora)*

Laurel (berry, leaf) *(Laurus nobilis)*

Myrtle *(Myrtus communis)*

Nutmeg (East Indian) *(Myristica fragrans)*

Star anise *(Illicium verum)*

MELANOMAS

Bergamot (expressed unrectified) *(Citrus bergamia)*

ESTROGEN-DEPENDENT CANCERS

Citronella *(Cymbopogon nardus, C. winterianus)*

Eucalyptus *(Eucalyptus globulus, E. maidenii, E. plenissima, E. polybractea, E. radiata, E. smithii)*

Fennel (bitter and sweet) *(Foeniculum vulgare)*

Lemongrass *(Cymbopogon flexuosus)*

Melissa (lemon balm) *(Melissa officinalis)*

Star anise *(Illicium verum)*

Verbena *(Aloysia triphylla, Lippia alba)*

Diabetes

Diabetes occurs when the pancreas does not produce enough insulin or the cells of the body do not respond to insulin appropriately. Insulin is a hormone that signals cells in the body to absorb glucose from the blood; the cells use glucose for energy. When insulin levels are insufficient or cells are resistant to insulin signaling, blood sugar levels rise. Diabetes, characterized by hyperglycemia (high blood sugar levels), excessive thirst, and overproduction of urine, results. There are three types:

+ **Type 1,** also referred to as juvenile or insulin-dependent diabetes, is systemic and occurs when the body fails to produce enough insulin. Type 1 requires insulin injections into the body to redress the balance.

✦ **Type 2,** also referred to as adult-onset diabetes, occurs when the body fails to respond to insulin appropriately. As the condition continues, a lack of insulin develops. Type 2 diabetes can be controlled through diet and is often triggered by excessive body weight and lack of exercise.

✦ **Gestational diabetes** occurs during pregnancy as a result of high blood glucose levels, even when there is no previous history of diabetes.

In some diabetics, circulation is poor, skin sensation may be altered, and the skin can become very fragile. The healing process can be very slow, particularly in the lower legs and feet. Bruising is also common.

Certain essential oils may produce a hypo- or hyperglycemic response; although this response mainly relates to oral intake, in the interest of caution, avoid topical use of the essential oils listed below.

Essential Oils with a Hypoglycemic Effect

Cinnamon bark *(Cinnamomum verum)*

Dill *(Anethum graveolens, A. sowa)*

Fennel *(Foeniculum vulgare)*

Geranium *(Pelargonium × asperum)*

Myrtle *(Myrtus communis, Backhousia anisata)*

Sage (Dalmatian) *(Salvia officinalis)*

Any essential oils containing citral (for example, lemongrass, may chang, melissa, palmarosa, lemon-scented tea tree, and lemon verbena)

Essential Oils with a Hyperglycemic Effect

Rosemary *(Rosmarinus officinalis)*

Essential Oils to Avoid in Type 1 (Insulin-Dependent) Diabetes

Black seed *(Nigella sativa)*

Cassia *(Cinnamomum cassia)*

Cinnamon bark *(Cinnamomum verum)*

Dill *(Anethum graveolens, A. sowa)*

Fennel (bitter, sweet) *(Foeniculum vulgare)*

Fenugreek *(Trigonella foenum-graecum)*

Geranium *(Pelargonium × asperum)*

Lemon basil *(Ocimum × citriodorum)*

Lemongrass *(Cymbopogon citratus, C. flexuosus)*

Lemon leaf (lemon petitgrain) *(Citrus × limon)*

Lemon-scented tea tree *(Leptospermum citratum)*

May chang *(Litsea cubeba)*

Melissa (Lemon Balm) *(Melissa officinalis)*

Myrtle (aniseed, honey, lemon) *(Backhousia anisata, Melaleuca teretifolia, Backhousia citriodora)*

Star anise *(Illicium verum)*

Turmeric (rhizome) *(Curcuma longa)*

Verbena *(Aloysia triphylla, Lippia alba)*

(Tisserand and Young 2014, 118)

Asthma

Asthma is a chronic inflammatory disease of the airways characterized by recurring episodes of airflow obstruction caused by bronchospasm. Common symptoms include coughing, wheezing, chest tightness, and shortness of breath. The majority of reported asthma cases are related to allergic rather than irritant reactions. Overexposure to environmental pollution is increasingly attributed to and cited as a causative factor in the rising reported incidence of asthma. However, there seems to be no evidence that pure essential oils cause either irritant or allergic asthma.

On the other hand, strongly scented perfumes containing synthetic scent molecules and odor fixatives, present alongside essential oils, and odors from powerfully scented flowers, such as hyacinth and lilac, do demonstrate potential for irritant or allergic responses capable of triggering allergic or irritant asthma. Absolutes should be considered in the same vein as perfumes in this instance.

While essential oils have not been found to *cause* asthma, they may still *trigger* an asthma attack because vaporized essential oils irritate the mucous membranes in the airways. Tisserand and Young (2014, 105–9) confirm that some essential oils do contain compounds that can cause eye and airway irritation, however, this can depend on the amount of oil inhaled and how long you are exposed to the compounds. They also observe that other essential oils and their components can have potential *anti-allergic* effects. For example, they remind us that chamazulene inhibits the formation of inflammatory prostaglandins and leukotriene B4, and therefore may have a therapeutic effect in calming allergic asthma or rhinitis. Deodar cedarwood (*Cedrus deodara*) has anti-inflammatory effects that may prevent histamine release (Tisserand and Young 2014, 238). English lavender essential oil, bergapten (found in expressed citrus oils such as bergamot, lime, and grapefruit as well as essential oils such as rue and angelica root), and eugenol (found in cinnamon, clove, and basil essential oils, and in small amounts in jasmine and rose absolute) also have antihistamine effects (105). They confirm that, while delta-3-carene, limonene, alpha-pinene, and beta-pinene are reported in isolation as irritants, there is also clinical data that suggests that these compounds, and essential oils containing them, may in fact be therapeutic when used to treat respiratory disease, especially in synergy with other components within an essential oil (109).

Those with a history of asthma (or other sensitivities or allergies to perfumes and other scented products) should use essential oils with caution, in moderation, in reduced amounts (0.5% to 1% dilution), alternating the types of essential oils and taking breaks occasionally.

Essential Oils That Seem Safe for Asthmatics (Applied Topically and in Moderation)

Chamomile, Roman *(Anthemis nobilis)*

Cypress *(Cupressus sempervirens)*

Frankincense *(Boswellia carterii, B. neglecta, B. sacra)*

Lavender, English *(Lavandula angustifolia)*

Mandarin *(Citrus reticulata)*

Peppermint *(Mentha × piperita)*

Petitgrain *(Citrus aurantium var. amara)*

Do not use or inhale essential oils during an asthma attack, and avoid direct inhalation of essential oils in general. For general immune and antihistamine support, apply essential oils topically in an ointment, oil, or cream chest rub.

ADDITIONAL MEDICAL CONDITIONS: ESSENTIAL OILS TO AVOID

MEDICAL CONDITION	CONTRAINDICATED ESSENTIAL OILS
Benign prostatic hyperplasia (BPH)	Lemongrass *(Cymbopogon flexuosus)*, lemon ironbark *(Eucalyptus staigeriana)*, lemon myrtle *(Backhousia citriodora)*, may chang *(Litsea cubeba)*, melissa *(Melissa officinalis)*
Cardiac fibrillation	Cornmint *(Mentha arvensis)*, peppermint *(Mentha × piperita)*
Fever	Annual wormwood *(Artemisia annua)*, balsamite (camphor chemotype) *(Chrysanthemum balsamita)*, camphor (white) *(Cinnamomun camphora)*, ho leaf (camphor/safrole chemotype) *(Cinnamomum camphora)*, hyssop *(Hyssopus officinalis)*, lavender cotton *(Santolina chamaecyparissus)*
Kidney disease	Indian dill *(Anethum sowa)*, parsley leaf and seed *(Petroselinum crispum)*
Liver disease	Indian dill *(anethum sowa)*, parsley leaf and seed *(Petroselinum crispum)*

Contraindications for Massage

Massage is a wonderful, nurturing, and remedial tool for well-being, with so many positive benefits beyond relaxation—for instance, improved muscle tone and suppleness, skin tone, and lymph-vascular circulation as well as positive parasympathetic stimulation and immune system support. However, there are certain conditions where the stimulating effect of massage is not advisable. If you have a cold or flu, or some other viral or bacterial infection, for example, your body's immune system will already be hard at work fighting these invaders. Massage can overstimulate the system and worsen a condition, and the toxins released from the muscle and skin tissues through massage can overload the body's excretory system. Massage can also, in the same way, exacerbate or spread an infection to other areas of the body. Viral and bacterial infections can also be contagious.

As a rule of thumb, do not massage if you or the other person has any infectious condition or condition you do not understand, has had recent surgery or an accident, or if you generally feel unwell or have any other doubt, for any reason, about whether you should proceed.

The lists below include a range of conditions—from those with absolute contraindication, that is, *no* massage at all, to those where massage can be applied with specific care and caution. This list includes both infectious and noninfectious conditions.

Conditions with *Absolute Contraindications* to Massage

Any infectious illness—for example, chickenpox, cirrhosis of the liver (if due to viral agent), diarrhea (if due to infection), German measles, influenza, laryngitis (if caused by infectious agent), measles, mumps, pharyngitis (if due to infection), pleurisy (if caused by infectious agent), ringworm, tonsillitis

Any acute condition

Appendicitis

Autoimmune disease (during flare-up)

Cardiac arrest

Cholecystitis (during flare-up)

Contact dermatitis (if widespread area is involved)

Embolism

Encephalitis

Fever

Gallstones (during gallbladder attack)

Gout (during acute phase)

Hemorrhage

Hepatitis (during acute phase)

Hives (during acute phase)

Hypertension (if not controlled by diet, exercise, and/or medication)

Intestinal obstruction

Jaundice

Lupus (during flare-up)

Meningitis

Migraine headache (during the migraine headache episode)

Mononucleosis

Multiple sclerosis (during flare-up)

Pancreatitis (if acute)

Pericarditis

Pneumonia (during acute phase)

Preeclampsia

Psychiatric diagnosis of manic depressive psychosis, schizophrenic psychosis, or paranoid conditions

Pulmonary embolism

Pyelonephritis

Rabies

Recent injury (wait seventy-two hours or until medical clearance is given)

Respiratory distress syndrome

Rheumatoid arthritis (during flare-up)

Scarlet fever

Scleroderma (during flare-up)

Tuberculosis

Conditions That Require *Medical Clearance* Prior to Massage

Acromegaly

Aneurysm

Arthritis

Atherosclerosis

Burns

Cancer

Cerebrovascular accident

Chronic obstructive pulmonary disease

Congestive heart failure

Coronary artery disease

Hemophilia

Hodgkin's disease

Kidney stones

Leukemia

Motor neuron disease

Multiple sclerosis

Myasthenia gravis

Nephrosis

Osteoporosis

Parkinson's disease

Peritonitis

Polycystic kidney disease

Pregnancy

Uremia

Conditions with *Localized Contraindications* for Massage

Abdominal diastasis (avoid abdomen)

Abnormal lumps (avoid area)

Acne vulgaris (avoid infected area)

Athlete's foot (avoid infected area)

Blister (avoid area)

Bruise (avoid area)

Carpal tunnel syndrome (avoid inflamed area)

Colitis (avoid abdomen)

Cretinism (avoid throat)

Crohn's disease (avoid abdomen)

Cystitis (avoid abdomen)

Decubitus ulcers (avoid ulcerated area)

Diverticular disease (avoid abdomen)

Folliculitis (avoid infected area)

Foreign objects embedded in the skin, such as glass, pencil lead, or
    metal (avoid area)

Furuncle/carbuncle (avoid infected area)

Goiter (avoid throat area)

Gouty arthritis (avoid infected area)

Grave's disease (avoid throat region and any enlarged lymph nodes)

Hernia, such as hiatal, femoral, inguinal, or umbilical (avoid herniated area)

Herpes simplex (avoid infected area)

Hypothyroidism (avoid throat area)

Impetigo (avoid infected area)

Irritable bowel syndrome (avoid abdomen)

Local inflammation (avoid inflamed area)

Onychomycosis (avoid infected area)

Open wounds (avoid wounded area)

Paronychia (avoid infected area)

Phlebitis (massage only lightly over the affected area)

Polyps (avoid abdomen)

Poison ivy, poison oak, or poison sumac (avoid affected area)

Seborrheic keratosis (avoid infected area)

Shingles (avoid infected area)

Spina bifida (avoid lumbosacral area)

Swollen lymph glands (avoid swollen area)

Thrombophlebitis (massage only lightly over the affected area; avoid inner thigh region)

Ulcers (avoid abdomen)

Unhealed burns and abrasions (avoid injured area)

Urinary incontinence (avoid abdomen)

Urinary tract infection (avoid abdomen)

Varicose veins (massage only lightly over the affected area)

Wart (avoid infected area)

Avoiding Interactions with Medications

Essential oils may complement certain medical treatments, but they must form part of a holistic treatment or care strategy, where all involved are able to make informed choices in the best interest of a positive outcome. Do not use essential oils for a condition already being treated with medication; chemicals within essential oils may compromise, exacerbate, or counteract the chemical actions of certain medications. Do not use essential oils while undergoing cancer treatment (radio- or chemotherapy), as these treatments heighten sensitivity to other chemicals, especially odorous chemicals, and compromise skin integrity, especially around treatment sites. Always check the cautions and contraindications of both conventional medications and essential oils before applying concurrently.

ESSENTIAL OILS TO AVOID
WITH CERTAIN MEDICATIONS

MEDICATION	CONTRAINDICATED ESSENTIAL OILS
Acetaminophen	**Oral ingestion** of anise *(Pimpinella anisum)*, basil *(Ocimum basilicum, O. tenuiflorum, O. × citriodorum, O. gratissimum)*, bay (West Indian) *(Pimenta racemosa var. racemosa)*, camphor *(Cinnamomum camphora)*, cinnamon (bark, leaf) *(Cinnamomum verum)*, clove (bud, leaf) *(Syzgium aromaticum)*, and fennel *(Foeniculum vulgare)*
Aspirin	**Oral ingestion** of allspice (berry, leaf) *(Pimenta dioica)*, bay (West Indian) *(Pimenta racemosa var. racemosa)*, cinnamon leaf *(Cinnamomum verum)*, clove (bud, leaf) *(Syzgium aromaticum)*, garlic *(Allium sativum)*
CYP2D6 substrates, including imipramine, amitriptyline, and codeine	**Topical application** of balsam poplar *(Populus balsmifera)*, **chamomile (German) *(Matricaria recutita)*,** sage *(Salvia officinalis, S. lavandulifolia)*, and yarrow *(Achillea millefolium)*; *Oral ingestion* of chaste tree *(Vitex agnus castus)*, cypress (blue) *(Callitris intratropica)*, jasmine sambac (absolute) *(Jasminum sambac)*, and sandalwood (W. Australian) *(Santalum spicatum)*
Meperedine	**Oral ingestion** of parsley (leaf, seed) *(Petroselinum sativum), and parsnip (Pastinaca sativa)*
Warfarin	**Oral and topical application** of sweet birch *(Betula lenta)* and wintergreen *(Gaultheria fragrantissima)*

Constituents within these oils may inhibit or potentiate the drug action. Please refer to Tisserand and Young's *Essential Oil Safety*, 2nd edition, for further information.

Special Considerations during Pregnancy

Caution must be observed during pregnancy to protect the developing fetus. Because essential oil molecules do enter the bloodstream, they may cross the placenta and potentially enter the bloodstream of the fetus. There is insufficient evidence regarding the full effect that certain essential oils or their chemical components may have on the central nervous system and brain of the developing fetus or, indeed, the mother's hormone balance and uterine tissue.

Opinion remains divided. Some texts provide advice about using essential oils during pregnancy, while others recommend that essential oils should be completely avoided.

Essential oils are highly concentrated potential sensitizers and irritants, and pregnancy can increase the propensity for sensitivity in some women. I recommend avoiding them during the first trimester of pregnancy. After the first trimester, essential oils may be diluted in vegetable/plant oil or lotions and applied through massage (avoiding the abdomen and breasts). Always ensure that you know the chemical properties and cautions and contra-indications associated with an essential oil before using it. Consult a professional aromatherapist, your midwife, or your primary-care physician for advice.

Essential Oils to Avoid during Pregnancy

Estrogen-like essential oils: clary sage *(Salvia sclarea)*, fennel *(Foeniculum vulgare)*, geranium *(Pelargonium × asperum)*, niaouli *(Melaleuca quinquenervia)*, rose otto *(Rosa × damascena, R. × centifolia)*, ylang ylang *(Cananga odorata)*

Strong emmenagogues: basil *(Ocimum basilicum, O. tenuiflorum, O. citriodorum, O. gratissimum)*, fennel (bitter, sweet) *(Foeniculum vulgare)*, hyssop (pinocamphone chemotype) *(Hyssopus officinalis)*, juniper berry *(Juniperus communis)*, marjoram *(Origanum marjorana)*, myrrh *(Commiphora myrrha)*, parsley (leaf, seed) *(Petroselinum crispum)*, rosemary *(Rosmarinus officinalis)*, sage *(Salvia officinalis, S. lavandulifolia)*

Others: aniseed (anise) *(Pimpinella anisum)*, anise (star) *(Illicium verum)*, carrot seed *(Daucus carota)*, cinnamon (leaf, bark) *(Cinnamomum verum)*, cypress (blue) *(Callitris intratropica)*, ho leaf (camphor chemotype) *(Cinnamomum camphora)*, lavender (Spanish) *(Lavandula stoechas)*, myrtle *(Myrtus communis)*, nutmeg *(Myristica fragrans)*, oregano *(Origanum vulgare, O. onites)*, thuja (northern white cedar) *(Thuja occidentalis)*, western red cedar *(Thuja plicata)*, yarrow (green) *(Achillea nobilis)*

Essential Oils Considered Safe during Pregnancy (in a 1% Blend)

Chamomile (Roman) *(Anthemis nobilis)*

Jasmine (Spanish) *(Jasminum grandiflorum)*

Mandarin *(Citrus reticulata)*

Neroli (bitter orange blossoms) *(Citrus × aurantium)*

Petitgrain (orange leaf) *(Citrus aurantium var. amara)*

Sandalwood (Indian and W. Australian) *(Santalum album, S. spicatum distilled)*

Ylang ylang *(Cananga odorata)*

Special Considerations for Children and the Elderly

Children and the very elderly require special consideration because they tend to be more sensitive and vulnerable to skin and organ damage, and they tend to have weaker immune systems and so may be more inclined to react to certain essential oils. In both cases the dose should be reduced to one-half to one-third of the dose for a healthy adult, depending on the size and age of the child or the condition of the elderly person. From the age of fifty-six onward, the skin becomes thinner and metabolism slows; however, many older people remain active, healthy, and robust and can continue to be treated as a healthy adult.

Do *not* use essential oils on babies under twelve weeks old. There is mixed opinion regarding the use of essential oils at all on babies that are less than eighteen months old or even toddlers under the age of three. There are essential oils that should definitely *never* be used on babies or children in any circumstance (see below). In general, for children, avoid using any essential oils that contain ketones, phenols, or aldehydes or have hormonal activity.

Never allow babies or children under the age of twelve to ingest essential oils. Do not apply essential oils neat (undiluted) to children's skin. In fact, do not use essential oils on a child's skin unless the child is over eighteen months old, the essential oils are known to be safe, and they are extremely diluted in an appropriate carrier medium. A safe dilution would be no more than 0.05 to 1 percent (1 or 2 drops of essential oil in 10 ml of vegetable/plant oil). Use no more than 1 or 2 drops of essential oil in one day, use occasionally, and do not use the same essential oil repeatedly.

Essential oils may also be vaporized environmentally (for example, chamomile, lavender, or mandarin can be vaporized in a child's room to ease restlessness and improve sleep). Other safe applications for children include the following:

Baths: 1 drop of essential oil diluted in 15 ml of vegetable oil, added to the bathwater; this can make the bath slippery, do not leave child unsupervised. Vaporizing or diffusing essential oils in the bathroom at bathtime can be very effective too, and may be preferable to adding diluted essential oils to bathwater.

Body massage: 1 or 2 drops of essential oil in 20 ml of vegetable/ plant oil, lotion, cream, or gel

Facial application: ½ to 1 drop of essential oil in 20 ml of vegetable/ plant oil, lotion, cream, or gel

Essential Oils to Avoid in Babies and Children

All herbaceous (e.g., marjoram, oregano, rosemary, thyme) and spicy essential oils

Fennel (bitter, sweet) *(Foeniculum vulgare)*

Hyssop *(Hyssopus officinalis)*

Juniper berry *(Juniperus communis)*

Star anise *(Illicium verum)*

Safe Essential Oils for Children*

Chamomile (Roman) *(Anthemis nobilis)* (at 0.025% = 1 drop in 20 ml)

Lavender (English) *(Lavandula angustifolia)*

Mandarin *(Citrus reticulata)*

Patchouli *(Pogostemom cablin)*

Sandalwood (Indian) *(Santalum album)*

---

*These essential oils are deemed safe for children only with the reduced dosage described on page 121.

Safe Essential Oils for the Elderly*

THE SERENITY ESSENTIAL OILS

Cajeput *(Melaleuca cajuputi)*

Carrot seed *(Daucus carota)*

Chamomile (German and Roman) *(Matricaria recutita, Anthemis nobilis)*

Cypress *(Cupressus sempervirens)*

Frankincense *(Boswellia carterii, B. sacra)*

Galbanum *(Ferula galbaniflua)*

Geranium *(Pelargonium graveolens, P. × asperum)*

Lavender (English) *(Lavandula angustifolia)*

Mandarin *(Citrus reticulata)*

Patchouli *(Pogostemon cablin)*

Petitgrain *(Citrus aurantium* var. *amara)*

Rose otto *(Rosa × centifolia, R. × damascena)*

Spikenard *(Nardostachys jatamansi, N. grandiflora)*

Tea tree *(Melaleuca alternifolia)*

Vetivert *(Vetiveria zizanioides)*

---

*These essential oils are deemed safe for the elderly only with the reduced dosage described on page 121.

Aromatherapy, when practiced within clearly defined and appropriate boundaries, provides a safe and very effective method of supporting and maintaining health and well-being. The psycho-emotional and immune-supporting properties of essential oils are especially valuable for treating stress and stress-related conditions, particularly because long-term stress can compromise the immune system. The physiological and psycho-emotional versatility of essential oils means that the boundaries of therapeutic application can overlap and/or become blurred.

When applying essential oils, users should keep in mind all the cautions and contraindications associated with the oils, as well as all the dynamics and potential negative interactions associated with various health conditions and medications. People who are using essential oils on their own, rather than under the care of a qualified provider, should refer to a professional health-care practitioner if they recognize "red flag" symptoms or if they persistently feel unwell.

The context in which aromatherapy is practiced will determine whether aromatherapists need complementary skills (e.g., a nursing qualification) or whether they work alongside other specialized health-care professionals. Professional collaboration across the health-care sector represents a truly universal health-care system, within which aromatherapy, as a practice of diligently using essential oils "to promote or improve human health, hygiene and well-being" (Tisserand n.d.), has a significant role to play.

Essential Oil Uses

Physiological

Immune Support
- Cajeput
- Carrot seed
- Cedarwood (Atlas)
- Chamomile (German)
- Clary sage
- Cypress
- Eucalyptus (globulus species)
- Frankincense
- Geranium
- Lavender (spike)
- Lemongrass
- Lime
- Mandarin

- Neroli
- Niaouli
- Orange (bitter)
- Petitgrain
- Sandalwood
- Tea tree
- Thyme
- Vetivert
- Skin & Wound Healing
- Cajeput*
- Calendula
- Cedarwood^
- Chamomile (German and Roman)
- Eucalyptus*
- Fennel (sweet)

- Galbanum
- Geranium
- Helichrysum
- Hyssop*
- Juniper*
- Lavender (English and spike)*
- Niaouli*
- Patchouli
- Rosemary*
- Sandalwood
- Tea tree
- Thyme*
- Yarrow
- Joint Pain
- Black pepper
- Cajeput*^

- Cedarwood (Atlas)^
- Chamomile (German and Roman)*
- Coriander*
- Ginger*
- Helichrysum
- Lavender (English and spike)*
- Marjoram
- Nutmeg*
- Pine*
- Thyme*
- Yarrow

Purification/Cleansing
- Effective against Microorganisms
- Cajeput++
- Cinnamon+++
- Clove+++
- Eucalyptus+++
- Geranium++
- Lavender (English)+++ (spike)+
- Lemon+
- Myrtle+++
- Niaouli++
- Oregano++++
- Peppermint+
- Pine+++
- Rosemary+
- Tea tree++++
- Thyme++++

- Antifungal
- Chamomile (Roman and German)
- Cinnamon bark
- Eucalyptus
- Lemon
- Lemongrass
- Myrrh
- Palmarosa
- Patchouli
- Tea tree
- Thyme
- Vetivert
- Antiseptic
- Bergamot^
- Chamomile (German)*
- Cinnamon*
- Clove*
- Eucalyptus*
- Garlic*
- Geranium^
- Lavender (English and spike)*^
- Lemon*
- Niaouli*

- Peppermint*
- Rosemary*
- Sandalwood*
- Thyme*
- Disinfectant
- Eucalyptus*
- Grapefruit
- Juniper*
- Lavender (English and spike)*
- Oregano
- Pine
- Sage*
- Thyme

Psycho-Emotional

Antidepressant
- Basil (Exotic)
- Chamomile (Roman)
- Chaste tree
- Clary sage
- Jasmine
- Lavender
- Melissa
- Neroli
- Scotch pine
- Thyme
- Ylang ylang

Nervous States
- Carrot seed
- Frankincense
- Lavender (English and spike)
- Marjoram (sweet)
- Neroli
- Spikenard
- Thyme
- Valerian
- Vetivert

Anxiety
- Basil
- Cedarwood
- Chamomile (German and Roman)
- Chaste tree
- Frankincense
- Helichrysum
- Lavender (English and spike)
- Mandarin
- Marjoram
- Neroli
- Patchouli
- Peppermint
- Petitgrain
- Thyme
- Valerian
- Vetivert
- Yarrow
- Ylang ylang

Hormone Stimulating
- REPRODUCTIVE
- Clary sage#
- Fennel#
- Geranium
- Niaouli#
- Rose
- Ylang ylang
- INSULIN
- Carrot seed
- Eucalyptus
- Fennel
- Geranium
- Lemon
- Thyme

Room Vaporizer
- Most essential oils, especially:
  - Fruits
  - Flowers
  - Woods
  - Resins

Aesthetic/Ambience

Single Oils
- ESSENTIAL OILS
- Jasmine
- Neroli
- Patchouli
- Rose
- Sandalwood
- Ylang ylang
- ABSOLUTES
- Jasmine
- Linden blossom
- Neroli
- Rose
- Violet

Perfume
Blends
- Basil
- Bergamot
- Black pepper
- Cajeput
- Cardamom
- Cedarwood
- Chamomile (German and Roman)
- Cinnamon
- Clary sage
- Clove
- Coriander
- Elemi
- Eucalyptus
- Fennel
- Frankincense
- Galbanum
- Geranium
- Ginger
- Grapefruit
- Jasmine
- Lavender (English and spike)
- Lemon
- Lemongrass
- Mandarin
- Melissa
- Myrtle
- Neroli
- Nutmeg
- Petitgrain
- Rose
- Rosemary
- Sandalwood
- Vanilla
- Vetivert

KEY

* = (Valnet/1980)   ^ = (Gattefossé/1937)   + = Strength   # = Estrogenlike

Serenity Essential Oils are listed in dark blue

4

Blending

Aligning Aesthetics and Therapeutics in Essential Oil Formulas

Our sense of smell is very subjective, influenced by a unique response inherent in our ancient intrinsic quest for survival and personal memory cues that we develop through day-to-day experience. What may smell pleasant to one person may be offensive to another, depending on his or her innate experience, perception, and even health (simply, we are attracted to what we need and repelled by what we do not). For example, consensus might be reached that a particular odor is very sweet; however, one person may describe that odor as *pleasantly* sweet, reminiscent of honey, while another person may describe it as *sickly* sweet, intense and unpleasant. Subjectively, both are right. Experiential interpretation and the language applied to describe odor differ from person to person. However, there are universally applied key terms attached to certain odor qualities that provide a basic common framework and point of reference.

Odors generally possess three observable traits:

- ✦ **Character or personality:** what the odor smells like (e.g., woody, fruity, sweet, haylike)
- ✦ **Intensity:** the strength of the odor (e.g., weak, strong, distinct)
- ✦ **Tenacity:** how long the odor remains present; its "staying power" (e.g., minutes, hours, days)

Together, these three traits comprise an essential oil's *fragrance profile.*

Essential oils are generally categorized into three broad groups according to their fragrance profile, the behavior of their predominant chemical components, and their volatility (rate of evaporation): These categories are called *notes,* in the musical sense (as in *tone, pitch, fast, slow, soft, loud, gentle, harmonious* and so on), to identify and acknowledge the multilayered, often complex qualities and nuances expressed by the various chemicals comprising an essential oil. Consider an orchestra harmonizing the sounds of various instruments to produce a melody— each chemical within an essential oil expresses its own unique tone, and each essential oil its own melody or harmony. When we blend essential oils, the aim is to create a particular tune, or story. In general, the notes break down as follows:

+ **Top notes:** quick, fast, rapid, and loud; the first scent to be experienced, and the first to fade; the most reactive; you can detect these notes when you first open an essential oil container.
+ **Middle notes:** harmonizers of the top and base notes, balancing the fast and slow qualities; the body of the scent; you can detect these notes thirty minutes after applying an essential oil formulation.
+ **Base notes:** gentle, soft, grounding, and heavy; the least volatile and most tenacious; the scent that lingers longest; you can experience these notes at *dry out* (when the essential oil formulation has dried on the skin, or a tissue), sixty minutes after application.

For ease of differentiation in this book, each category is attributed a color: red represents top notes, blue the middle notes, and green the base notes.

These are broad categories. Essential oils are complex. Each essential oil will express a range of top, middle, and base note qualities within its chemical mixture. Some essential oils teeter between or overlap categories. Categorization sometimes differs between authors. The following chart, however, offers a useful guide (see pages 128–29).

BLEND TYPES

Essential oil blending tends to fall into two categories:

+ **Aesthetic:** employing the hedonistic, psycho-emotional, social qualities of essential oils
+ **Therapeutic:** employing the psycho-emotional, physiological qualities of essential oils

Whether used as an aesthetic formulation or therapeutic remedy, essential oil blends are developed to be pleasing to the recipient, and in this sense there is inevitably an overlay between the therapeutic and aesthetic qualities of essential oils. There are very real differences, however, as outlined below.

Aesthetic Blends

A perfumer will often mix numerous odors in varying quantities to create a multifaceted blend of subtle nuances and tones that can be marketed as a themed or signature perfume. For example, Chanel No. 5 contains, among several other natural and synthetic ingredients, bergamot, neroli, rose, gardenia, jasmine, and vetivert; Paco Rabanne pour Homme contains, among other ingredients, citrus oils, lavender, clary sage, and cedarwood; 4711 Eau de Cologne contains lemon, lime, bergamot, tangerine, bitter orange, and so on. Although containing pure essential oils, perfumes also contain absolutes, concretes, and synthetically derived odorant chemicals, which may add tone to the scent dynamic or act as fixatives to stabilize the fragrance, lending tenacity to the perfume. Indeed, commercial perfumes can contain up to three hundred different natural and synthetic aromatic substances.

Each essential oil has its own scent profile, expressing a particular personality with various traits: masculine or feminine, uplifting, invigorating, calming, herbaceous, floral, woody, volatile, light, illusive, viscous, heavy, lingering, and so on. Like characters in a play, these personalities are selectively blended to purposefully tell a story within a specific ambience, mood, or theme: youthful, mature, fun, sensual, passionate, nighttime, daytime, exotic, a garden in summer,

ESSENTIAL OIL CHARACTERISTICS

You will note that some oils appear in more than one category. These oils are identified with an asterisk. They are listed first with their primary categorization and then in italics for the category they move toward. For example, cypress presents as a middle note but moves toward a base note, where it is represented in italics; petitgrain is a top note but may move toward a middle note depending on its fragrance profile. Serenity Essential Oils are indicated in boldface.

CHARACTERISTIC	TOP NOTE	MIDDLE NOTE	BASE NOTE
Type of oil	Lemon and other citrus fruits; leaves	Herbs; flowering tops	Resins, woods, roots, blossoms
Volatility rate (on a scale of 1 to 100)	1 to 14	15 to 60	61 to 100
Evaporation rate	0 to 30 minutes	Up to 8 hours	Usually 12 to 24 hours, possibly a week, sometimes longer
Action	Fastest	Moderate	Slowest
General fragrance characteristic	Sharpish	Round	Heavy
Dry-out odor quality	Fresh, distinctive, cluster of odors; obvious, light, and potentially intense due to rapid evaporation	Lingering traces of top notes; heart of the bouquet; softer edges	Lingering traces of middle notes; faint, faded, subtle, nondescript; heavy, tenacious residue
Therapeutic effects	Uplifting, stimulating, revitalizing; aids memory and brain function	Balancing, harmonizing, rejuvenating	Relaxing, grounding, sedating, calming
Skin penetration	½ to 1 hour	2 to 3 hours	4 to 6 hours or more
May support/ease (general indications)	Extreme lethargy, melancholy, lack of interest, apathy, acute depression	Bodily functions, metabolism, digestion, menstruation, circulation (blood pressure)	Nervous, erratic, flighty, or hyperactive behavior; anxiety; chronic and/or long-standing conditions; the elderly
Essential oils	Basil	Black pepper	Benzoin
	Bergamot	**Carrot seed**	Cedarwood*
	Cajeput	*Cedarwood**	Cinnamon bark

ESSENTIAL OIL CHARACTERISTICS (*continued*)

CHARACTERISTIC	TOP NOTE	MIDDLE NOTE	BASE NOTE
	Caraway	Chamomile (German and Roman)	Clove
	Citronella	Clary sage*	Cypress*
	Clary sage*	Cypress*	Frankincense*
	Eucalyptus	Fennel*	Helichrysum
	Fennel*	Frankincense*	Jasmine
	Galbanum	Geranium	Myrrh
	Ginger	Juniper	Neroli*
	Grapefruit	Lavender (English and spike)	Patchouli
	Lemon	Marjoram	Rose otto*
	Marjoram	Neroli*	Rose absolute
	Lemongrass	Oregano	Sandalwood
	Mandarin	Palmarosa*	Spikenard*
	May chang	Peppermint*	Valerian
	Niaouli	Petitgrain*	Vetivert
	Nutmeg	Pine	Ylang ylang*
	Orange (sweet)	Rose otto*	
	Palmarosa*	Rosemary	
	Peppermint*	Rosewood*	
	Petitgrain*	Spikenard*	
	Rosewood*	Thyme (white and red)*	
	Tea tree	Ylang ylang*	
	Thyme (white and red)*		

a meadow in spring, blossom in a Mediterranean orchard, and so on.

Essential oils have been used in perfumes since ancient times to enhance attractiveness, stimulate a "feel good" factor, mask unpleasant smells, and more. Thanks to their versatility and wide range of characteristics, they have also been used in other products, such as foods and household products, to enhance or aid in synthetically mimicking a particular odor or flavor or to obscure less pleasant–smelling constituents, with the added benefit being that their antimicrobial qualities can extend a product's shelf life. (See the list of products containing essential oils below.) Blending essential oils to create a pleasant, effective perfume at its best is indeed a work of art driven by an intuitive, creative process. And, as with all expressions of art, the artist, perfumer, or creator inevitably projects through the lens of their own perception and the perceiver observes through theirs.

Products Containing Essential Oils

Air fresheners	Laundry detergent
Alcohol	Lotions and creams
Animal feed	Meat products
Antiseptics	Mouthwash
Baked goods	Nasal sprays
Beverages (especially teas)	Ointments
Candles	Paint
Canned food	Paper
Confectionary	Perfumery (cologne, aftershave)
Convenience foods	Pharmaceuticals
Cosmetics and toiletries	Preservatives
Cough syrups	Printing ink
Dentistry products	Rubber manufacturing
Detergents	Soap
Disinfectants	Soft drinks
Fabric softener	Stomachics/laxatives
Food and drink flavorings	Textile products
Food colorings	Throat lozenges
Gargles	Tobacco
Glue/adhesives	Toothpaste
Ice cream	Veterinary products
Insect repellents/insecticides	

Therapeutic Blends

Aromatherapeutic blends, while also aiming to please, usually comprise only two to four individual essential oils and are less intricate and complex in their design than perfumes. In aromatherapeutic blending, specific chemical actions and therapeutic qualities guide the selection of essential oils, the aim being to hone, accentuate, and support a specific quality to create an effective remedy. For example, mandarin (*Citrus reticulata*), English lavender (*Lavandula angustifolia*) and rose otto (*Rosa* × *centifolia*) may be blended to promote a sense of feeling calm yet uplifted, to aid in relaxation, or as an antidote to anxiety.

I have noticed that mandarin essential oil often triggers memories or images of warm summer days, rose otto seems to instill a sense of luxury and self-worth, and lavender a sense of feeling safe and calm; then, as the more volatile components leave the odor, the layers beneath initiate other responses. The major chemical constituent groups (monoterpenes, esters, and alcohols) found within these three essential oils are attributed with antiseptic, antiviral, anti-inflammatory, and immune-stimulating qualities, among others. So, as well as acting as an emotionally uplifting and grounding remedy, a blend of the three would also provide preventive wellness and immune support. In this way, essential oils affect different elements of need at one and the same time. Buckle (2007), observing this multidynamic quality, noted that a client attracted, for example, to the odor of lemongrass for its sedative effects may incidentally also benefit at the same time from its antifungal properties when that essential oil is added to a soothing footbath originally prescribed for relaxation.

BLENDING ESSENTIAL OILS

Because essential oils are used extensively in so many of the products that we use every day, our memory associations may get in the way when we first smell a particular essential oil's scent. For example, a scent may remind us of furniture polish, toilet cleaner, disinfectant, different types of foods, and so on. Equally, because essential oils are concentrated, their aromas can be overwhelming: however, unlike synthetic perfumes and commercial odorizers, which contain chemical fixatives, the scent of essential oils naturally fades.

When learning to create your own blends of essential oils, it seems sensible to start by focusing on a small group of them (perhaps up to six), and to smell and use these essential oils until their qualities become familiar and any other memory association is diluted or transcended. Then you may gradually introduce other essential oils, experimenting in the same way, taking the time to learn about their qualities, and in so doing to considerately develop your repertoire. Once you are familiar with individual essential oils, blending them together becomes easier.

As described previously, each chemical within an essential oil expresses its own unique tone or note, and every essential oil expresses its own distinctive melodic harmony or tune based on its chemical arrangement. As such, essential oils and their chemical components are loosely categorized into three broad categories: top, middle, and base. Top notes are the most volatile (the ones you immediately notice, and the first to leave) and base notes are the least volatile (the ones that linger behind after the others have left). Over time an essential oil's original signature melody alters; the orchestra dismantles until all that is left is a lingering ensemble ambling melodiously into the dusky hours of evening. The following tables will aid your essential oil selections. You can decide whether you want each oil to perform solo or as part of a duet, trio, quartet, or, in the case of perfumes, a band or orchestra. The dry-out scent, or lingering ensemble, is as significant as the initial full-bodied scent—the mellow evening melody impression made by the first performance of the day—both need to be pleasing.

When blending essential oils, it is advisable to include at least one middle note in all blends to maintain a link between the fast (top note) and slow (base note) elements. Start by blending two or three oils and experiment with the ratios. For example, you might combine 3 drops of a base note essential oil, 2 drops of a middle note essential oil, and 1 drop of a top note essential oil to create a relaxing and sedating blend. Then, using the same three essential oils, you might combine 2 drops of the base note, 3 drops of the middle note, and 1 drop of the top note and compare the two blends. Blending essential oils to create a pleasing scent is a subjective process. Enjoy your journey of discovery and ignite the creative artist within you using the following charts and exercises as a starting guide.

BASIC SCENT CHARACTERIZATIONS AND EXAMPLES OF ESSENTIAL OILS WITH THESE CHARACTERISTICS

Serenity Essential Oils are indicated in boldface.

CHARACTERIZATION	SCENT CORRELATION	ESSENTIAL OIL EXAMPLE
Agrestic	Like meadows, forests, moss, soils of the earth	**Galbanum,** oakmoss
Balsamic	Warm, woody, sweet and vanilla-like	Benzoin absolute, **frankincense,** Peru balsam, vanilla
Burnt	Smoky, scorched	Undertones of cedarwood, **vetivert**
Camphoraceous	Like camphor	**Cajeput,** eucalyptus, **spike lavender,** marjoram, **patchouli,** sage (Dalmatian), **tea tree**
Citrus	Like citrus fruits	Citronella, bergamot and **mandarin** (and other citrus essential oils), lemongrass
Clean	Cool, fresh, sharp notes	Mint, **patchouli**
Coniferous	Like pine, with tones of turpentine	**Cypress,** pine
Dry	Dusty, powdery, not sweet	Middle notes of clove bud; base notes of **galbanum, patchouli,** and rosemary; middle and base notes of **petitgrain,** juniper berry, black pepper
Earthy	Like rain-moistened earth	Base notes of **galbanum,** middle notes of **carrot seed** and **patchouli, vetivert**
Floral	Like fragrant flowers, whether a single flower or a bouquet	**Chamomile (Roman), geranium,** jasmine, neroli, **rose otto,** ylang ylang
Fresh	Citrusy green top notes and green-herbaceous middle notes, cool and summerlike, newly bloomed	Minty essential oils, **mandarin** and other citrus oils

CHARACTERIZATION	SCENT CORRELATION	ESSENTIAL OIL EXAMPLE
Fruity	Like various edible fruits	**Chamomile (Roman), frankincense,** middle notes of jasmine, **mandarin,** orange, and ylang ylang
Green	Like crushed green leaves	**Galbanum,** violet absolute
Herbaceous	Like culinary herbs or a bouquet garni	Basil and other herb oils; middle notes of bergamot, **carrot seed,** and neroli; **chamomile (Roman); lavender;** top notes of **patchouli**
Light	Delicate, ethereal, not distinctive	Dry out notes of basil, **lavender, mandarin**
Medicinal	Medicine-like	Juniper, myrrh, middle notes of **tea tree,** thyme, ylang ylang
Minty	Like crushed mint leaves	**Geranium,** mint, peppermint
Mushroomy	Musty, damp, and fungal-like	Middle notes of jasmine and **lavender (English)**
Pithy	Like the pith of citrus fruit after it's removed from the fruit	Dry-out notes of bergamot and **mandarin** (and other citrus oils)
Resinous	Like fragrant resins	**Frankincense,** myrrh
Rich	Persistently sweet and mellow; sickly in excess	Clove bud, **geranium, patchouli, rose otto**
Sharp	Piquant, penetrating	Top notes of **galbanum,** lemon, and **mandarin**
Spicy	Like culinary spices	Clove, cinnamon, middle notes in **rose otto** and **spikenard**
Sweet	Suggestive of sweetness of taste	Top notes of basil, **chamomile (German), geranium,** fennel, and **mandarin;** middle notes of may chang
Woody	Like exotic woods	**Carrot seed,** cedarwood, cypress, **petitgrain**

(Adapted from Williams 2006, 125)

ODOR INTENSITY RANGE
OF SERENITY ESSENTIAL OILS

ODOR INTENSITY	ESSENTIAL OIL
Extremely high	Galbanum
High	Chamomile (German and Roman), frankincense, patchouli, rose otto, spikenard, tea tree, vetivert
Fairly high	Cajeput, carrot seed, geranium
Medium	Cypress, lavender (English and spike), petitgrain
Low	Mandarin

Note: Essential oils with high odor intensity will dominate a blend unless used in moderation.

SERENITY ESSENTIAL OIL SCENT PROFILES

Each essential oil typically has a primary role to play—top note, middle note, or base note—in a blend's scent, and that's how the essential oils in this table are organized, but in addition, each oil has its own top, middle, and base notes as described below.

ESSENTIAL OIL	TOP NOTES (FIRST IMPRESSION)	MIDDLE/BODY NOTES (AT 30 MINUTES)	BASE/DRY-OUT NOTES (AT 60 MINUTES)
Cajeput	Mild, sweet, fresh, and clean but camphoraceous, with menthol; softly metallic	Detectable but faint residue of top notes; camphoraceous, soft, clean, sweet, and herbaceous, with greeny-woody tones	Very faintly herbaceous
Galbanum	Powerful, fresh, sharp, green, balsamic, slightly sweet, and herbaceous with earthy-woody undertones	Green, coniferous, balsamic, and agrestic	Dry, earthy, and spicy
Mandarin, green	Initial but fleeting sharp notes, fresh, warm, fruity, intense, deep, sweet, and softly citrusy	Fading, faintly fruity, tangeriney, soft, round, and light	Faded, very faint, barely detectable, slightly herbaceous-fruity, pithy

SERENITY ESSENTIAL OIL SCENT PROFILES (*continued*)

ESSENTIAL OIL	TOP NOTES (FIRST IMPRESSION)	MIDDLE/BODY NOTES (AT 30 MINUTES)	BASE/DRY-OUT NOTES (AT 60 MINUTES)
Petitgrain	Fresh and floral, woody, citrusy; similar tones to neroli	Dry, floral, herbaceous, woody	Dry, herbaceous
Tea tree	Strongly camphoraceous; metallic	Warm, camphoraceous, spicy, medicinal, and metallic	Faint, little characteristic
Carrot seed	Dry, "carroty," slightly sweet, woody, earthy, mushroomy, and slightly herbaceous	Earthy, "carroty," peppery, and herbaceous	Very faded but detectable; earthy, "carroty," and peppery
Chamomile (German)	Sweet, warm, herbaceous, and fruity	Sweet, herbaceous, and hay-like, with soft agrestic notes	Warm and tobacco-like
Chamomile (Roman)	Sweet, fruity, and herbaceous, with soft floral undertones	Warm, herbaceous, and somewhat fruity	Warm, herbaceous, and tealike
Cypress	Fresh, woody-coniferous, and camphoraceous, with green notes	Coniferous and balsamic	Sweet and balsamic
Geranium	Rich, floral, roselike, sweet, and minty	Roselike, minty notes, with a hint of lemon and greens	Green and roselike
Lavender (English)	Fresh, floral, and slightly fruity	Herbaceous, floral, and slightly woody with mild camphoraceous tones	Faint, soft herbaceous
Lavender (spike)	Fresh and strongly camphoraceous	Camphoraceous, herbaceous, and woody	Faint herbaceous and woody
Frankincense	Fresh, lemony-fruity, green, and resinous	Resinous balsamic, slightly turpentine-like, woody, with citrusy-sweet tones	Lingering woody, slightly citrusy, balsamic-herbaceous

ESSENTIAL OIL	TOP NOTES (FIRST IMPRESSION)	MIDDLE/BODY NOTES (AT 30 MINUTES)	BASE/DRY-OUT NOTES (AT 60 MINUTES)
Patchouli	Sweet, rich, herbaceous, and balsamic	Sweet, earthy, slightly camphoraceous, spicy, mossy-woody, and balsamic	Tenacious, dry, woody, balsamic, and spicy
Rose otto	Powerful, complex, sweet, fresh, highly floral and beeswax-like	Rich, waxy, floral, and spicy (clove-like)	Tenacious, soft, warm and floral notes
Rose absolute	Rich, intense, fresh, warm, deeply floral, almost intoxicating	Floral, fresh, sweet, warm, with citrusy tones	Tenacious lingering floral-citrusy notes
Spikenard	Very sweet, intense, and fresh pea–like, with tones of fresh grass; slightly woody	Less intense and delicately woody, with undertones of spice, fresh pea, and hay	Sweet, with pea and hay notes; lingering
Vetivert	Sweet, complex, earthy, and burnt/smokey-woody	Rich, heavy, woody, earthy, and balsamic	Very tenacious, woody and earthy

(Adapted from Williams 2006; Watts 2001)

Therapeutic Blending: Getting Started

The following chart groups essential oils into plant types—trees, flowers, herbs, and so on. Within each type, essential oils are further grouped according to their botanical family. Blending essential oils from the same botanical family can enhance positive synergy. This is a guide to assist your initial selection. Always select an essential oil based on its individual chemical and therapeutic profile and then match complementary essential oils that will support these qualities to create a potent blend. Serenity Essential Oils are highlighted with boldface in the lists below. Absolutes such as oakmoss and hyacinth are also included. Remember that absolutes are prone to cause sensitization and irritation.

FLOWERS	TREES	HERBS	SPICE/SEED
Asteraceae (Compositae)	Cupressaceae	Labiatae (Lamiaceae)	Apiaceae (Umbelliferae)
Chamomile	Cade juniper	Basil	Angelica
(German, Roman,	Cedarwood	Calamintha	Aniseed
Maroc, English)	**Cypress**	Hyssop	Asafoetida
Calendula officinalis	Juniper	Marjoram	Caraway
Costus	**Lauraceae**	Melissa	**Carrot seed**
Helichrysum	Bay laurel	Mint	Celery seed
Lavender cotton	Camphor	Oregano	Coriander
Tagetes minuta	Cinnamon	Peppermint	Cumin
Tarragon	May chang	**Patchouli**	Dill
Yarrow	(*Litsea cubeba*)	Rosemary	Fennel
Violaceae	Rosewood	Sage	**Galbanum**
Violet	Sassafras	Clary sage	Lovage
	Ravensara	Thyme	**Malvaceae**
	Myrtaceae	**Verbenaceae**	Ambrette seed
	Allspice	Lemon verbena	**Myristicaceae**
	West Indian bay		Mace
	Cajeput		Nutmeg
	Eucalyptus		**Lauraceae**
	Myrtle		Cinnamon
	Niaouli		**Zingiberaceae**
	Tea tree		Cardamom
	Pinaceae (Abietaceae)		Ginger
	Canadian balsam		Turmeric
	Cedarwood atlas		
	Silver fir tree		
	Pine		
	Spruce		
	Turpentine		
	Fabaceae (Leguminosae)		
	Balsam (copaiba, Peru, tolu)		
	Cassie		
	Petitgrain (citrus)		
	Santalaceae		
	Sandalwood		
	Zygophyllaceae		
	Guaiacwood		

FLOWERS/ BLOSSOMS	TREES/RESINOUS	GRASS	FRUITS
Annonaceae	Burseraceae	Poaceae (Gramineae)	Rutaceae
Cananga	Frankincense	Citronella	Amyris
Ylang ylang	Linaloe	Lemongrass	Bergamot
Oleaceae	Myrrh	Palmarosa	Grapefruit
Jasmine	Opopanax	Vetivert	Lemon
Liliaceae	West Indian birch		Lime
Hyacinth	**Dipterocarpaceae**		Mandarin
Rosaceae	Borneol		Orange (bitter,
Rose (cabbage,	Gurjun balsam		sweet)
damask, maroc)			**Piperaceae**
Rutaceae			Black pepper
Neroli (orange			Cubeba
blossom)			
FLOWERS/HERB	**SHRUBS/HERB**	**ROOTS**	**FUNGI (LICHEN)**
Geraniaceae	Cistaceae	Valerianaceae	Parmeliaceae
Geranium	Cistus	Spikenard	Oakmoss
(Bulgarian, rose)	Labdanum	Valerian	
Labiatae (Lamiaceae)	Star anise (Chinese, Japanese)	**Zingiberaceae**	
Lavender	**Liliaceae**	Ginger	
Lavendin	Hyacinth		

SERENITY ESSENTIAL OILS
THAT BLEND WELL TOGETHER

Cajeput	Lavender (English and spike), petigrain, rose otto
Galbanum	Geranium, lavender (English and spike)
Mandarin	Carrot seed, cypress, frankincense, geranium, patchouli, petitgrain, tea tree
Petitgrain	Geranium, lavender (English and spike), mandarin
Tea tree	Geranium, lavender (English and spike), mandarin
Carrot seed	Geranium, lavender (English and spike), mandarin
Chamomile (German)	Geranium, lavender (English and spike), patchouli, rose otto
Chamomile (Roman)	Cypress, geranium, lavender (English and spike), rose otto
Cypress	Chamomile (Roman), lavender (English and spike), mandarin, spikenard
Geranium	Carrot seed, chamomile (Roman), frankincense, galbanum, lavender (English and spike), mandarin, patchouli, petitgrain, rose otto, spikenard, tea tree
Lavender (English and spike)	All Serenity Essential Oils
Frankincense	Geranium, lavender (English and spike), mandarin, spikenard, vetivert
Patchouli	Geranium, lavender (English and spike), mandarin, rose otto, spikenard, vetivert
Rose otto	Most Serenity Essential Oils, especially chamomile (German and Roman), geranium, lavender (English and spike), patchouli, spikenard, vetivert
Spikenard	Cypress, frankincense, geranium, lavender (English and spike), patchouli, rose otto, vetivert
Vetivert	Frankincense, lavender (English and spike), patchouli, rose otto, spikenard

PROTOCOLS FOR FORMULATING
ESSENTIAL OIL BLENDS

Blending begins with making a comprehensive assessment of the fragrance of an essential oil, from initial impression to dry out. Only once you are deeply familiar with the qualities and properties of the scent

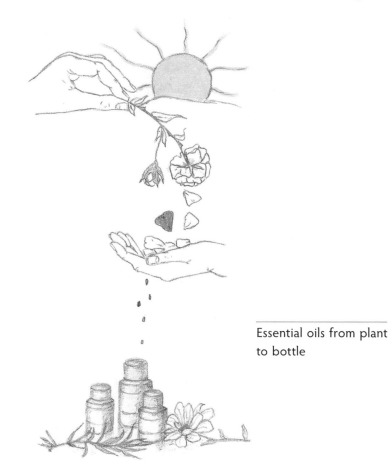

Essential oils from plant
to bottle

can you begin to consider how to blend that essential oil with others to formulate a therapeutic or aesthetic blend.

The following three exercises lay out protocols for assessing an essential oil's odor and formulating blends. To complete these exercises, you will need the following equipment:

+ Smelling strips (you can make these yourself by cutting thin strips of blotting paper; the dipping end should be pointed to allow insertion into the hole in a dropper cap) or tissues

+ Pen

+ Notepaper

+ Freshly ground coffee or coffee beans (if you are assessing more than one essential oil)

✦ The essential oils whose scent you would like to assess (assess no more than six at a time)

Note: Do not wear your own perfume or strongly scented deodorants during this exercise. Make sure your clothing does not have a strong scent of laundry detergent or fabric softener.

◊ Exercise 1: Becoming Familiar with Individual Essential Oils

There are two ways to generally assess essential oil odors: one immediate, instinctive, and reactive, the other controlled, deliberate, and responsive. Both, to an extent, are underpinned by intuition. Smelling an essential oil straight from the bottle (immediate) gives an instant but incomplete impression. In order to fully appreciate the characteristic depths and dynamics of the scent, it is best to release an essential oil from its bottle onto a tissue or smelling strip, thus allowing full vaporization to occur and revealing the true layers and depths of its personality.

Preparing Your Equipment and Work Area

1. Ensure that your work area has adequate ventilation (an open window will suffice).
2. Ensure that your work area has handwashing facilities and soap close by.
3. Ensure that a first-aid kit containing an eyebath is available.
4. Cleanse all work surfaces.
5. Set out a glass of fresh drinking water.
6. Place two or three spoonfuls of freshly ground coffee (or coffee beans) in a cup or small container (to smell between smelling essential oils).
7. Set out the essential oils you will be assessing.
8. Write the name of each essential oil being assessed on a smelling strip or tissue.
9. List the essential oils to be assessed on your notepaper. Use the following worksheet as a guide.

ESSENTIAL OIL	VISCOSITY	COLOR	TOP NOTES (INITIAL ODOR IMPRESSION)	MIDDLE NOTES (ODOR AT 30 MINUTES)	DRY OUT (ODOR AT 60 MINUTES)
Mandarin, green (Citrus reticulata)					
Chamomile, German (Matricaria recutita)					
Frankincense (Boswellia carterii)					
Spikenard (Nardostachys jatamansi)					

Assessing the Scent of Essential Oils

1. Remove the lid from an essential oil bottle. Dip the pointed end of your smelling strip into the hole in the dropper cap, or place 1 drop of essential oil on the smelling strip or tissue. Replace the essential oil bottle lid immediately.

2. Hold the smelling strip or tissue a hand's width below your nose, gently moving or waving the tissue backward and forward. Inhale the evaporating essential oil odor, taking long, slow breaths through your nose.

3. Notice how the odor feels as it passes through your nasal cavity, down your throat, and into your lungs. Can you "taste" it as you inhale? In which part of your nose or throat do you register the odor?

4. Assess the characteristics of the scent. What do you smell immediately? What is prominent?

5. Assess your own response to the scent. Does the odor remind you of anything? Does it invoke particular thoughts or memories? What are you feeling as you smell the odor?

6. Hold the tissue away while you take a clear breath; perhaps sip some water. Then repeat steps 2 through 5, this time noticing the depth or layers of scent (that is, the undertones) behind the initial odor you observed.

7. Repeat this process (steps 2 through 6) for two to three minutes. Notice if the odor changes during this period.

8. Note the color of the essential oil; does the essential oil stain or color the strip or tissue, or is it colorless? Note the viscosity; how thick or thin is the essential oil?

9. Write your observations on your prepared paper, noting the time.

10. Let the strip sit for thirty minutes, then repeat the exercise, making your notes as before. Now you are assessing the middle notes.

11. Let the strip sit for another thirty minutes, then repeat the exercise again, making your notes as before. Now you are assessing the dry-out or base notes. (Note: Ideally, essential oils should be left to oxidize (evaporate) on the strip or tissue over a period of at least twenty-four hours to get a true impression of the dry-out odor.)

Guidelines for Assessing the Scent of Several Essential Oils

- Sip some fresh water and smell the freshly ground coffee (or coffee beans) after smelling each essential oil. Take a few clear breaths before commencing with the next essential oil.
- Do not smell more than three or four essential oils consecutively. If you are assessing more oils than that, divide them into smaller groups, and take a thirty-minute (preferably longer) "breathing space" between each group. Leave the room if possible.

When you are finished with your assessment, your notepaper will contain a detailed record of the essential oils you worked with. It might look something like the following:

ESSENTIAL OIL	VISCOSITY	COLOR	TOP NOTES (INITIAL ODOR IMPRESSION)	MIDDLE NOTES (ODOR AT 30 MINUTES)	DRY OUT (ODOR AT 60 MINUTES)
Mandarin, green (Citrus reticulata)	Thin liquid; drops quickly from the bottle	Light olive-green stain on the tissue; it fades slightly as the essential oil evaporates, leaving a soft yellow-green stain	Fresh, fruity, intense, deep, sweet, and softly citrusy; like mandarin peel	Fading, faintly fruity, tangeriney, soft, and round	Faded, very faint, barely detectable, slightly herbaceous-fruity
Chamomile, German (Matricaria recutita)	Thin liquid; drops quickly from the bottle	Deep green-blue stain on the tissue; it fades, becoming more green-yellow with subtle blue	Sweet, warm, herbaceous, and fruity; sickly, slightly unpleasant	Sweet, herbaceous, and haylike	Warm and tobacco-like; lingering
Frankincense (Boswellia carterii)	Thin liquid; drops quickly from the bottle	Clear wet mark on the tissue; liquid in the bottle is slightly yellow; the visual evidence fades, leaving no stain, but the aroma remains on the tissue	Fresh, lemony-fruity, green, and resinous	Resinous balsamic, slightly turpentine-like, woody, with citrusy-sweet citrus tones	Lingering woody, slightly citrusy, balsamic-herbaceous
Spikenard (Nardostachys jatamansi)	Moderately viscous, thick appearance; drops slowly from the bottle	Pale amber, slightly bluish-green tint; the color fades, leaving a yellowy-cream stain on the tissue	Very sweet, intense, and fresh pea–like, with tones of fresh grass; slightly woody	Less intense and delicately woody, with undertones of spice, fresh pea, and hay	Sweet, with pea and hay notes; lingering

Safety Considerations

- If your skin comes into direct contact with essential oils, wash the affected area immediately.
- To avoid irritation of the mucous membranes, do not hold the smelling strip or tissue too close to your nose when inhaling the odor; this is especially important if you are assessing several essential oils consecutively.
- If you accidentally transfer essential oil into your eyes (e.g., touching your eyes with your fingers), rinse your eyes *immediately* with warm water until you are sure the essential oil has been washed out. If your eyes continue to feel irritated, seek medical attention promptly.
- Stop the exercise if you feel dizzy, become nauseous, or begin to get a headache.
- Do not engage in this exercise if you are pregnant or feel generally unwell.
- Do not engage in this exercise if you have not eaten for a long period of time.
- If you are taking medication for any reason, ensure that it will not have any negative interactions with the essential oils you will be assessing.
- Clean up any essential oil spillages immediately.

◊ Exercise 2: Creating a Therapeutic Blend

Once you have completed the first exercise, you will be ready to experiment with blending essential oils to create pleasing remedies. Use the observations you made in the first exercise to guide your choice of essential oil combinations. Begin by selecting the primary essential oil (the "signature" oil) of the blend. This will be an oil that strongly expresses the theme of your choice (antidepressant, anti-anxiety, uplifting, calming, et cetera), and it may be a top, middle, or base note. Then selectively add essential oils to enhance the therapeutic properties and odor profile of your signature oil to create your personalized remedy.

For therapeutic blends, combine no more than three or four individual essential oils. If you are creating a blend that you would like to have enduring effects (for example, a therapeutic perfume), ensure that you include more base and middle notes than top notes to enhance the tenacity of the scent.

For example, you may select frankincense as your signature essential oil to complement meditation, yoga, or other relaxation techniques. Frankincense essential oil has a green, resinous-woody middle note and subtle earthy odor;

it appears to inspire deeper breathing and a sense of calm. To support the therapeutic properties and scent profile of frankincense, which is, as identified above, a base note, you might blend it with Roman chamomile, a middle note, and green mandarin, a top note, thus harmonizing your odor profile. As well as aiding relaxation, this blend will relieve restlessness and inability to sleep (especially for children), soothe anxiety, alleviate mild depression, and will generally ground, balance, and uplift mood and emotion.

It is important to be aware of the evolution of a scent as the lighter tones evaporate. Those tones that linger behind will ultimately contribute to the body and the lingering dry-out tones of the scent and require as much consideration when formulating blends as the fresh, initial scent. As the top notes leave the blend of essential oils, those notes that remain must still maintain a pleasing combined aroma.

Preparing Your Equipment and Work Area

1. Ensure that your work area has adequate ventilation (an open window will suffice).
2. Ensure that your work area has handwashing facilities and soap close by.
3. Ensure that a first-aid kit containing an eyebath is available.
4. Cleanse all work surfaces.
5. Set out a glass of fresh drinking water.
6. Place two or three spoonfuls of freshly ground coffee (or coffee beans) in a cup or small container (to smell between smelling essential oils).
7. Clearly identify the theme or reason for your blend. For example, you might intend to formulate a blend that is uplifting or calming, or a blend to complement meditation or relaxation, or a blend to ease insomnia, and so on.
8. Select candidates for the blend's signature essential oil—ones that meet the intention behind the theme of the blend. Then select possible complementary essential oils that support and harmonize with the signature oil both therapeutically and aesthetically. Set out all of these essential oils on your work surface to be assessed.
9. Write the name of each essential oil being assessed on a smelling strip or tissue.
10. List the essential oils to be assessed on your notepaper. Use the worksheet on page 148 as a guide.

As explained earlier, your signature essential oil may be a top, middle, or base note. In the example below, I use petitgrain and mandarin. Both are top notes. However, as previously established, petitgrain also moves toward a middle note. Petitgrain and citrus fruit oils complement and enhance each other's qualities, and I often combine them in a blend to potentiate their uplifting qualities. The complementary top, middle, and base note columns below list examples of essential oils that support petitgrain and mandarin to achieve an uplifting yet grounding and balancing blend that may alleviate feelings of depression.

SIGNATURE THEME	SIGNATURE ESSENTIAL OIL	COMPLEMENTARY TOP NOTE	COMPLEMENTARY MIDDLE NOTE	COMPLEMENTARY BASE NOTE	CHOSEN BLEND(S)
Remedy for mild depression	Petitgrain (Citrus aurantium var. amara) Mandarin, green (Citrus reticulata)	Galbanum (Ferula galbaniflua)	Roman chamomile (Anthemis nobilis) Cypress (Cupressus sempervirens) English lavender (Lavandula angustifolia)	Rose (Rosa x centifolia) Spikenard (Nardostachys jatamansi) Frankincense (Boswellia sacra)	

Assessing the Scent of Essential Oils

Follow the instructions given in Exercise 1 (see pages 143–44), retaining each strip.

Blending Your Selected Essential Oils

1. Select your signature essential oil smelling strip.
2. Select the smelling strips of the complementary essential oils that you think will blend well with your signature essential oil.
3. Hold the smelling strips together a hand's width from your nose and inhale.
4. Experiment, changing the combinations of smelling strips until you are satisfied with the potential of the combined odor.
5. Note your essential oil blend selections. Use the worksheet on page 149 as a guide.
6. Choose your method of application (see chapter 7).

Once you have selected your essential oils, you can then experiment with ratios. For example, you can tune the scent and therapeutic profile of your blend by adjusting the number of drops of each essential oil you add together. So, for Blend 1 below, I might add 1 drop of rose, 2 drops of cypress, and 2 drops of petitgrain. Rose is very intense, so 1 drop is often sufficient in a blend. For Blend 2, I might add 1 drop of spikenard, 2 drops of lavender, 1 drop of galbanum, and 1 drop of mandarin. For Blend 3, I might add 2 drops of frankincense, 1 drop of Roman chamomile, and 2 drops of mandarin. My choice, in this example, very simply, depends on whether I want my blend to be predominantly balancing, uplifting, or grounding. Depending on your need and chosen method of application, you can then add these essential oils to vegetable oil, cream, or lotion for body application, or add to water in an environmental diffuser (see chapter 7). This is a basic guide. Preparations for more serious conditions require deeper understanding of essential oil chemistry, physiology, and pathology.

SIGNATURE THEME	SIGNATURE ESSENTIAL OIL	COMPLEMENTARY TOP NOTE	COMPLEMENTARY MIDDLE NOTE	COMPLEMENTARY BASE NOTE	CHOSEN BLEND(S)
Remedy for mild depression	Petigrain *(Citrus aurantium var. amara)* Mandarin, green *(Citrus reticulata)*	Galbanum *(Ferula galbaniflua)*	Roman chamomile *(Anthemis nobilis)* Cypress *(Cupressus sempervirens)* English Lavender *(Lavandula angustifolia)*	Rose *(Rosa × centifolia)* Spikenard *(Nardostachys jatamansi)* Frankincense *(Boswellia sacra)*	Blend 1: Petitgrain Cypress Rose Blend 2: Mandarin Galbanum Lavender Spikenard Blend 3: Mandarin Roman chamomile Frankincense

The Therapeutic Blending Guide Record on the following page suggests how you can record your blends and your selected methods of use each time you create a new remedy. This will allow you to create a catalog that will provide a reminder and serve as a future point of reference. (It's easy to forget small, specific details in the blur of everyday things; making notes is a useful way to anchor information.) You could also add a section to note the outcome of your blend and application method (the scent, the effectiveness of the medium, how often and how long you applied it, what changes you might make to the blend next time, and so on). The same principles apply to the Aesthetic Blending Guide Record (pages 153–54).

THERAPEUTIC BLENDING GUIDE RECORD (SAMPLE)

Signature Condition				
Secondary Condition (if applicable)				

		Note
Signature Essential Oil		

Supporting Essential Oils (no more than three)	Top Note	Middle Note	Base Note

Carrier Medium/ Method of Application	☐ Vegetable oil(s) (for massage or skin care) ☐ Cream ☐ Lotion ☐ Ointment ☐ Aloe Vera Gel ☐ Compress ☐ Roller Bottle (therapeutic perfume) ☐ Face Mask ☐ Nasal Inhaler ☐ Environmental Diffuser ☐ Other _____

Essential Oil Blend		Number of Drops
	1. _____	
	2. _____	
	3. _____	
	4. _____	
	Total Drops	
		Amount
	Carrier medium _____	

◊ Exercise 3: Creating an Aesthetic Blend

To create an aesthetic perfume, first decide on the signature of your blend—that is, the theme you want to portray (masculine, feminine, invigorating, sensual, et cetera). Then decide how you want to convey your signature theme—that is, which qualities will express the theme (e.g., woody, floral, fruity, spicy, summery, et cetera). Select essential oils that fit into your signature fragrance "picture," following the guidance set out in Exercise 2.

Preparing Your Equipment and Work Area

Follow the instructions given in Exercise 2 (see page 147), setting out the essential oils you've selected as candidates for an aesthetic blend and recording their names on smelling strips and on a worksheet (use the one on page 148 as a guide).

Assessing the Scent of Essential Oils

Follow the instructions given in Exercise 1 (see pages 143–44), retaining each strip.

Blending Your Selected Essential Oils

1. Select your signature essential oil smelling strip.
2. Select the smelling strips of the complementary essential oils that you think will blend well with your signature essential oil.
3. Hold the smelling strips together a hand's width from your nose and inhale.
4. Experiment, changing the combinations of smelling strips until you find a blend that portrays the mood, image, or impression you envisage (in doing so, you may discover dynamics you had not imagined or previously considered).

   Remember that top notes give the first impression but are flighty and leave quickly. Base notes tend to hold back or slow down the release of the more volatile components and thus lend blends some tenacity or staying power; base notes generally linger long after the top and middle notes have evaporated. And the dry-out odor requires as much consideration as the immediate odor impact when creating a blend.
5. Note your essential oil selections. Use the worksheet on page 149 as a guide.
6. Begin building your perfume picture with base notes, then add middle notes, then top notes, using more base notes and middle notes than top notes (see the figure on page 152). It's best to limit the number of different essential oils (or absolutes) you use initially. This way you can try out different melodies, and experiment with different harmonies, before creating your symphony! Add essential oils carefully, drop by drop; it is easy to add a drop to your blend, but once added, it is impossible to remove, so take your time.

   Start with up to six different oils, and, as in exercise 2, experiment with your essential oil drop ratios to tune your perfume. Note the number of drops of each essential oil you add to your blend, and note each time how this alters the scent profile. (Thus, you will have a record of how your perfume structure develops as you build in different scent nuances.) Observe the collective scent of the base notes, then how this begins to alter as you add middle notes, then top notes.

7. Once you are happy with your blend, add it to your chosen carrier medium—e.g., vegetable or jojoba oil, cream or ointment, or alcohol (ethanol or vodka). Note how doing this may change the scent of your blend slightly; you may want to add drops or adjust your essential oil ratio to accommodate this.

8. Once you are happy with your final scent, tightly secure the container's lid and leave your perfume to stand for twenty-four hours in a cool dark place, thus allowing the mixture time to settle. Alcohol evaporates rapidly and can cause skin irritation; if you use alcohol as a base for your perfume, apply it to your clothes rather than your skin. Oil- or cream-based perfumes last longer and also protect skin from the potential irritant effects of essential oils. (Please refer to chapter 7 for information about using perfume roller bottles and making ointments, along with various other methods of application.)

9. Over the following days and weeks, monitor the developing fragrance of the blend. Some essential oils, like chamomile, rose, and vetivert, are intense right out of the bottle and will initially dominate a blend. They will require fewer drops, but their dry-out odor may be less intense, which will change the odor dynamic. Experiment.

Note: Remember, do not apply essential oils neat to your skin. Rather, apply neat essential oils to clothes or tissues, or blend in a carrier medium such as jojoba oil, coconut oil, or alcohol.

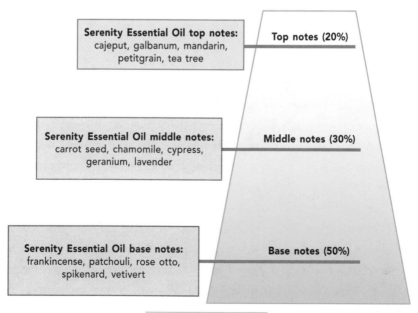

Serenity Essential Oil top notes: cajeput, galbanum, mandarin, petitgrain, tea tree — Top notes (20%)

Serenity Essential Oil middle notes: carrot seed, chamomile, cypress, geranium, lavender — Middle notes (30%)

Serenity Essential Oil base notes: frankincense, patchouli, rose otto, spikenard, vetivert — Base notes (50%)

Aesthetic blend ratios

Blending 153

AESTHETIC BLENDING GUIDE RECORD (EXAMPLE)

As previously established, the sense of and response to an odor is extremely personal and is influenced by numerous factors, such as the time of day, season, scent memories, state of health, and so on at the time of perception. The recipe below provides an example of the blending process; the scent created may be liked or disliked or received with indifference depending on a person's frame of reference.

FLORAL GROUNDING AND UPLIFTING BLEND

Signature essential oil: Rose

Signature of Blend	☑ Feminine ☐ Masculine ☑ Uplifting ☐ Invigorating ☐ Attractant ☐ Calm but strong ☐ Other _____
Odor Theme	☐ Woody ☐ Spicy ☑ Floral ☐ Fruity/Citrus ☐ Other _____
Carrier Medium	☐ Vegetable oil ☐ Cream ☐ Lotion ☐ Perfume ointment ☑ Perfume (roller bottle – jojoba oil) ☐ Perfume (alcohol-based) ☐ Bath Oil ☐ Other_____ **Quantity** _10 ml_

NO. OF OILS	ESSENTIAL OIL	DROP RECIPE/ SEQUENCE OF ADDING DROPS	TOTAL NUMBER OF DROPS	COMMENT/ ODOR DEVELOPMENT
BASE NOTES				
1	Rose	2 + 1 + 1	4	Floral, sweet, deep, intense
2	Spikenard	1	1	Fresh, woody, earthy, floral
3	Patchouli	1	1	Earthy, woody, slightly floral
MIDDLE NOTES				
1	Geranium	1	1	Slightly sweet, earthy, dry, slightly floral
TOP NOTES				
1	Petigrain (top to middle note)	2	2	Citrusy, slightly acidic, woody undertones
2	Madarin	1	1	Mossy, mellow,citrussy
Total drops in the Blend			10	Final blend: floral, rosy, slightly citrussy with earthy-mossy undertones

AESTHETIC BLENDING GUIDE RECORD (SAMPLE)

TITLE OF BLEND:

Signature essential oil:

Signature of Blend	☐ Feminine ☐ Masculine ☐ Uplifting ☐ Invigorating ☐ Attractant ☐ Calm but strong ☐ Other _____
Odor Theme	☐ Woody ☐ Spicy ☐ Floral ☐ Fruity/Citrus ☐ Other _____
Carrier Medium	☐ Vegetable oil ☐ Cream ☐ Lotion ☐ Perfume ointment ☐ Perfume (roller bottle – jojoba oil) ☐ Perfume (alcohol-based) ☐ Bath Oil ☐ Other_____ **Quantity** _____

NO. OF OILS	ESSENTIAL OIL	DROP RECIPE/ SEQUENCE OF ADDING DROPS	TOTAL NUMBER OF DROPS	COMMENT/ ODOR DEVELOPMENT
BASE NOTES				
MIDDLE NOTES				
TOP NOTES				

5

Building Connections

*Exploring Subtle Energies
and Dynamics*

This chapter will focus specifically on the energies and subtle dynamics of Serenity Essential Oils. These oils are among the safest and also most effective, and as you will discover, they provide a spectrum of valuable effects and influences. They also readily complement other modalities and practices of holistic health care and well-being.

COLOR

Electromagnetic energy radiates from the sun and takes just over eight minutes to travel the distance to Earth. Upon reaching the atmosphere surrounding the planet, these rays of electromagnetic energy are attenuated, primarily by ozone and water vapor, reducing the intensity of their flux, and are scattered by molecules of air and aerosols.

There are many types of electromagnetic energy or radiation. All are similar in form but with differing rates of flux (how much of something is flowing through a surface in a given amount of time). Infrared waves (heat), X rays, visible light, and radio waves are all types of electromagnetic radiation. The frequency of their oscillation ranges from high to low and from short to long wave.

Cosmic rays   **Radium rays**

Gamma rays

     Hard X rays
     Grenz rays

X rays

     Erythemal rays
     Fluorescent rays

Ultraviolet light

Magenta	*higher frequency*
Violet (Blue)	
Blue (Cyan)	
Turquoise	
Green	
Yellow	
Orange	
Red	*lower frequency*

Visible light

     Radiant heat rays
     Photographic rays

Infrared rays   **FM radio, TV, radar, shortwave band,**
Radio waves   **commercial broadcasting**

Color and the electromagnetic spectrum

How We Perceive Color

Everything we see depends on our sensory perception of reflected light. Each color expressed in the spectrum of light that is visible to humans resonates at a different frequency or wavelength; we perceive different wavelengths of light as different colors. Light waves reflect off objects in our spatial environment; when those waves reach our eyes, color, shade, and shadow (the obstruction of light) give visual depth, contour, shape, texture, differentiation, position, and a sense of space and orientation.

There are two types of photo, or light, receptors in the retina of the eye: rods and cones. Rods are responsible for vision at low levels of light, do not mediate color vision, and have low spatial acuity; they are sensitive to light intensity and are responsible for night vision. Cones are active at higher levels of light, are capable of color vision, and have high spatial acuity; they are responsible for daytime vision.

There are three types of cones within the eye: one sensitive to short wavelengths (blue light), another to middle wavelengths (green light), and another to long wavelengths (red light). When these photoreceptors are stimulated by light wavelengths, they send neural signals to the brain, which interprets and labels the wavelengths as colors. As a resonant vibrational frequency, color is also detected and responded to by other senses and aspects of the body.

Colors of Light vs. Colors of Pigments

Colored light is reflective. Pigment color, on the other hand, is absorptive. When light waves hit objects or substances of a different density, some wavelengths are absorbed by the pigment matter on the surface of the object; other wavelengths are reflected from the pigment matter, and those are the wavelengths that we perceive.

+ **Colors of light:** The three primary colors of light are red, blue and green. When blended together in equal combination they create the appearance of white light.
+ **Colors of pigment:** The three primary colors of pigment are yellow, cyan and magenta, which when combined create the appearance of black pigment—the absence of light.

Combining primary colors creates new colors, known as secondary colors. The primary colors of light are the secondary colors of pigments, and the primary colors of pigments are the secondary colors of light.

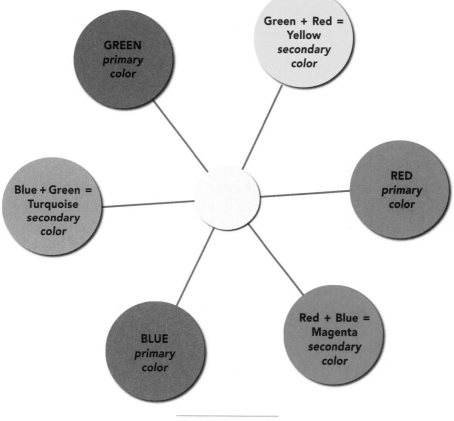

The colors of light

Color Therapy for Energetic Healing

Color plays a large role in the therapeutic use of essential oils, gemstones, and chakras in energetic healing. Gemstones and essential oils have pigment colors. Chakras, on the other hand, resonate at the frequency of light. Each chakra resonates with the full color spectrum, but one color dominates over the others. So, for example, red dominates the base chakra, yellow dominates the solar plexus chakra, and blue dominates the throat chakra. Ideally, each chakra resonates in harmony with

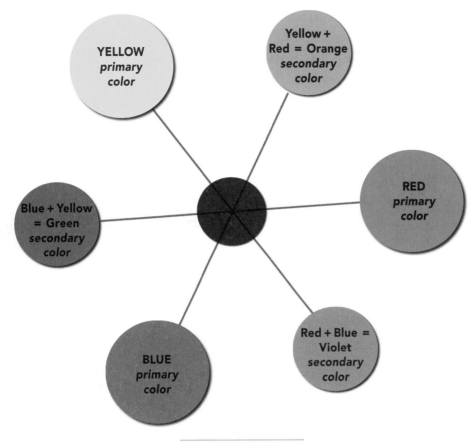

The colors of pigment

the other chakras with equal strength. However, this state is in constant flux, and sometimes one chakra is weaker or more dominant than the others, which creates imbalance. The aim of therapy is to rebalance and harmonize the chakra's vibration by applying light or pigment color to help strengthen or unblock the affected chakra to bring it back into balance with the rest.

Pigment colors (gemstones and essential oils) do not resonate at the same frequency as colored light (chakras). This can be partly addressed by combining a pigment color with its opposite color (which is, confusingly enough, also called its *complementary* color). These paired gemstones resonate similarly to colored light, and when applied in a healing context can help maintain balance between the chakras. They are further enhanced by the use of essential oils, and vice versa. For example, cypress essential oil might be selected to counterbalance a lack of self-confidence and feelings of anxiety or nervousness before an important job interview or performance, where clarity of thought and the ability to answer questions spontaneously with calm assertiveness is important. To optimize the desired qualities of this essential oil, the gemstone citrine (color: yellow) may be applied along with its complementary opposite gemstone, amethyst (color: violet/purple). The citrine would be applied to the solar plexus chakra, which resonates with the color yellow, while the amethyst would be applied to the crown chakra. Both gemstones could also be placed together in your hand or worn as jewelry, such as a pendant.

In trio, Serenity Essential Oils, color, and gemstones create a potent combination, which may be further potentiated when massage is also included.

GEMSTONES

The term *gemstone* is used here to mean crystals and minerals, and also to portray a sense of their preciousness in terms of their healing and balancing qualities and, of course, their beauty. The information presented here regarding gemstones draws on their complementary qualities in relation to the subtle dynamics of essential oils. But we only touch upon the full capacities of gemstones here. Gemstone healing represents a complete system unto itself.

Gemstones are gentle in their action and safe to use alongside other therapies. Generally speaking, they are energizing, cleansing, clearing, and protective, and they can amplify the qualities of other remedies, such as flower essences and essential oils, and provide complementary elements that may support their qualities. Gemstones will not change a person's inherent intrinsic tendencies, but they may influence and support inner potential through rebalancing (increasing and decreasing) electromagnetic energy within the body. They are also mediums of transference for thoughts, intentions, and healing energy.

Gemstones and essential oils do not have exactly equal or parallel qualities; each have their own special values. However, there are certain common aspects that tentatively bring them together—the resonant influence of color, for example, being one. When carefully matched, each can enhance the potency of the other. Of course, as with essential oils, it is also possible to create a null or antisynergistic effect by putting too many dynamics into play at once. Therefore, I focus on a small select group of gemstones and generally match one primary gemstone and one essential oil to each chakra and associated color, which I find sufficient. I call this selection of gemstones, totaling nine, the Serenity Gemstones. (There are seven chakras, but the extra two gemstones— rose quartz and lapis lazuli—have influences bridging across chakras.)

QUALITIES OF THE SERENITY GEMSTONES

See the table on pages 168–70 for a listing of the chakras, essential oils, and other qualities associated with these gemstones.

GEMSTONE	COLOR	SPIRITUAL EFFECTS	MENTAL EFFECTS	EMOTIONAL EFFECTS	PHYSICAL EFFECTS	APPLICATION
Jasper	Red (but also found in brown, yellow, sandy colored, and green)	Stimulates a warriorlike nature. Helps us pursue and achieve goals with determination (red is the most dynamic, yellow the most calm, and green the most balancing).	Stimulates uprightness and honesty toward others and self. Helps us come to terms with and get a grip on tasks, even unpleasant ones. Stimulates the imagination. Helps us transform ideas into actions.	Imbues courage, readiness for action, determination, willpower (red), endurance (yellow), forthrightness, and ability to protect ourselves (and others) (green).	Stimulates circulation and flow of energy (red). Strengthens immune system (yellow), detoxifying and anti-inflammatory (green). Indicated for sexual, digestive and intestinal problems. Supports resistance to environmental stress (pollution, toxins, radiation).	Worn or laid in contact with the skin

QUALITIES OF THE SERENITY GEMSTONES (*continued*)

GEMSTONE	COLOR	SPIRITUAL EFFECTS	MENTAL EFFECTS	EMOTIONAL EFFECTS	PHYSICAL EFFECTS	APPLICATION
Carnelian	Orange (but also found in red, yellow and brown)	Promotes steadfastness, Encourages a spirit of community. Supports our willingness to help, to be idealistic, and our zealousness for a good cause.	Stimulates our facility to problem-solve speedily and pragmatically. Supports the conclusion of actions and a sense of realism in the face of confusion.	Bestows steadfastness and courage (everyday courage to overcome and face difficulties). Uplifts emotions.	Stimulates the absorption of vitamins, minerals, and nutrients in the small intestine. Alleviates rheumatism. Stimulates metabolism.	Worn or laid in contact with the skin.
Citrine	Yellow	Encourages individuality, self-confidence, and the courage to face and enjoy life. Encourages the desire for variety, new experiences, and self-realization.	Supports the "digestion" of impressions and ability to understand and support ourselves, as well as the ability to draw rapid conclusions.	Bestows joie de vivre. Helps us overcome depression and ties to oppressive influences. Encourages self-expression and extroversion.	Stimulates digestion and the processes of the stomach, spleen, and pancreas. Alleviates early-stage diabetes. Fortifies the nerves. Warming.	Worn in contact with the skin or used as environmental support for meditation.
Aventurine	Green	Reveals personal happiness/unhappiness. Fortifies self-determination and individuality. Stimulates dreaming; makes dreams come true.	Bestows a multitude of ideas and enthusiasm, yet encourages tolerance and acceptance of others' ideas and suggestions (balance).	Enhances relaxation, regeneration, and recovery. Helps us get to sleep. Encourages patience; calms anger and annoyance.	Encourages regeneration of the heart. Stimulates fat metabolism and lowers cholesterol levels (supports the heart). Anti-inflammatory. Alleviates skin disease, eruptions, and allergies. Fortifies connective tissues. Alleviates pain.	Worn as a pendant or laid on relevant parts of the body.

GEMSTONE	COLOR	SPIRITUAL EFFECTS	MENTAL EFFECTS	EMOTIONAL EFFECTS	PHYSICAL EFFECTS	APPLICATION
Rose Quartz	Pink	Encourages gentleness but firmness (not giving in but awareness of the capacity of a gentle, soft nature to overcome a hard, strong one). Encourages helpfulness, openness, and the desire for a pleasant ambience.	Liberates us from worry, helps us discriminate between sympathy and antipathy. Draws our attention to the fulfillment of elementary needs.	Imparts empathy and sensitivity— sometimes oversensitivity. Encourages balanced self-love, a strong heart, romance, and the ability to love.	Stimulates blood circulation in the tissues, fortifies the heart and sexual organs, helps with sexual problems, and encourages fertility.	Worn as a pendant or laid on relevant parts of the body, or used as environmental support for meditation.
Aquamarine	Green to light blue	Encourages spiritual growth, foresightedness, clairvoyant qualities. Aids us in being upright, goal-orientated, dynamic, persistent, and successful.	Clears confusion, stimulates orderliness, and helps us bring unfinished business to a conclusion.	Bestows light-heartedness and a happy, relaxed disposition (particularly due to all things we have undertaken progressing quickly and smoothly).	Harmonizes the pituitary gland and thyroid gland, thus regulating growth and hormone balance. Improves near- or far-sightedness. Calms overreactive immune system, thus helping with autoimmune diseases and allergies, especially hay fever.	Worn as a pendant or laid on relevant parts of the body.
Lapis lazuli	Deep blue	Bestows wisdom and honesty and reveals personal inner truth. Aids personal liberation from compromise and holding back.	Encourages self-awareness, dignity, honesty, and uprightness. Aids us in conveying our feelings and emotions; gives us voice.	Aids acceptance of and ability to face truth, while not negating personal views and opinions. Helps to contain conflict.	Aids healing of problems affecting the neck, larynx, and vocal cords (especially if originating from repressed anger). Regulates function of the thyroid gland.	Worn as a pendant or laid on relevant parts of the body, particularly the throat (just above the clavicle) or the forehead.

QUALITIES OF THE SERENITY GEMSTONES (*continued*)

GEMSTONE	COLOR	SPIRITUAL EFFECTS	MENTAL EFFECTS	EMOTIONAL EFFECTS	PHYSICAL EFFECTS	APPLICATION
Amethyst	Violet/ purple	Encourages constant spiritual wakefulness, a sense of spirituality, and insight into the reality of the spirit. Imbues us with a sense of justice, and the ability to judge. Inspires honesty and uprightness. Helps quiet the mind during meditation, and aids us in finding deep inner peace and wisdom.	Encourages sobriety and awareness. Helps us face up to all experiences, even unpleasant ones. Encourages us to consciously deal with perceptions, leading to heightened concentration and effective thinking and action. Encourages us to overcome blocks, uncontrolled mechanisms, and addictive behavior.	Helps in sadness and grief, lending support in coming to terms with loss. Clarifies inner world of images and dreams (placed under pillow, stimulates dreaming). Stimulates inspiration and intuition.	Helps relieve pain and tension, especially headaches. Assists with injuries, bruising, and swellings. Helps with nervous complaints, diseases of the lungs and respiratory tract, skin blemishes, and intestinal complaints. Encourages reabsorption of water.	Worn as a pendant, laid on relevant parts of the body, used as environmental support for meditation, or placed under the pillow to help us understand our dreams.
Sugilite	Violet	Helps us maintain our own point of view and live in accord with our own inner truth without deflection, either via pressure or persuasion.	Helps us deal with and overcome, conflicts without unnecessary compromise, finding solutions based on agreement, without disadvantage to either party.	Strengthens our ability to face up to unpleasant things. Dissolves inner tension and alleviates sorrow, grief, fears, and paranoia.	Has a harmonizing effect on the nerves and brain. Alleviates severe pain. Helps with epilepsy, dyslexia, and motor disturbances.	Worn as a pendant, laid on relevant parts of the body (especially areas of pain), or used as environmental support for meditation.

(Gienger 2004; Gerber 2001)

Of course, both gemstones and essential oils are multidynamic, so there is inevitably movement across the boundary between one chakra, color, or essential oil and another. An example of this is my choice of aquamarine as one of the primary gemstones for the throat chakra, in addition to the deep blue lapis lazuli. Aquamarine's qualities harmonize the thyroid and pituitary glands. Its gentle iridescent blue influences the throat chakra, and its green the adjacent heart chakra. In the context of the way that I apply gemstones, the qualities of aquamarine complement those of the deep green-blue German chamomile essential oil. As German chamomile oxidizes, its color becomes more deeply blue and less green; aquamarine is its perfect partner. The green in both the gemstone and the essential oil links to the heart chakra, so the voice (from the throat chakra) can "speak from the heart." The blue encourages honesty and openness, helps us overcome fear and find inner courage, and aids us in expressing and giving voice to our feelings. Among other therapeutic indications, both the essential oil and the gemstone also aid conditions that affect the upper chest, throat, and mouth.

Michael Gienger discusses the healing power of crystals in depth in his fascinating and informative book *Crystal Power, Crystal Healing*, which I recommend for those who want to further explore this subject.

THE CHAKRAS

The chakras are energy vortices, or portals, situated at major nerve plexuses and glandular centers of the endocrine system (for example, the pituitary, thyroid, adrenal, pancreas, and reproductive glands). As we learned earlier, the endocrine system regulates hormones, metabolism, growth, and affects almost every organ, including the brain and central nervous system, and cell in the body. The seven major chakras are located from the base of the spine to the top of the head, with several related minor chakras spread throughout the body. Each chakra resonates at a particular frequency, expressed as color, sound, and a particular life-force condition. Each chakra is associated with particular organs, which resonate at a similar frequency. For example, the fifth chakra (to elaborate the previous example) influences the major glands and structures within the throat and neck area, such as the mouth, vocal chords, trachea, cervical vertebrae, and thyroid and parathyroid glands, and is associated with the parasympathetic nervous system. This chakra is associated with communication and self-expression and giving voice to feelings and emotions. In an ideal state each chakra resonates at its optimal frequency, in harmony with the others; this is expressed within the body as a state of wellness and well-being. This harmony can be disrupted for various reasons (emotional or physical stress or trauma, for example). As you can see, this is a vast subject unto itself. Richard Gerber, in his fascinating book *Vibrational Medicine,* explains this phenomenon in much greater depth than I can afford here. My aim is to demonstrate how essential oils can be applied to support and balance the major chakras and their functions, as demonstrated in the illustration and charts that follow.

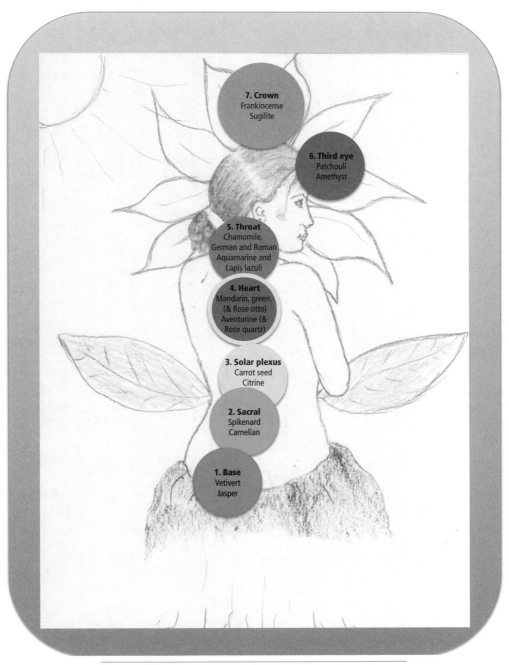

Chakras and key Serenity Essential Oils and Gemstones

THE CHAKRAS: CONNECTIONS AND ASSOCIATIONS

CHAKRA	LOCATION	ASSOCIATED PHYSIOLOGICAL SYSTEM	PSYCHO-SPIRITUAL/EMOTIONAL ATTRIBUTES	COLOR	ASSOCIATED GEMSTONES	ASSOCIATED SERENITY ESSENTIAL OILS
(1) Base or root (Muladhara)	Base of the spine	Reproductive	Ability to protect oneself and others, "best self," courage, endurance, forthrightness, honesty, life force, instincts, patience, readiness for action, determination, sense of feeling connected to the earth and grounded, stability, transformation of ideas into action, ability to be warriorlike, willpower	Red	Red jasper; also amber (red) bloodstone, garnet, obsidian, ruby, tourmaline (black)	Vetivert; also frankincense, rose absolute/otto, spikenard
(2) Sacral (Svadhishthana)	Just below the navel	Genito-urinary	Courage to overcome and face difficulties, creativity, endurance, idealism, new ideas, passion, pragmatism, realism, sexual attractiveness, problem solving, steadfastness, strength, vitality, willingness to help and inspire others, zealousness	Orange	Carnelian; also amber, calcite, fluorite (yellow), jasper (yellow), sunstone, tree agate	Spikenard; also carrot seed, patchouli, rose absolute/otto, vetivert
(3) Solar plexus (Manipura)	Just below the rib cage	Digestive	Action, balance, courage to face and enjoy life, "digestion" of impressions, humor, individuality, joy for life, laughter, new experiences, personal power, self-confidence, self-expression, self-realization, spontaneity, warmth	Yellow	Citrine; also amber, calcite, gold, tiger's eye, topaz (gold)	Carrot seed; also chamomile (Roman), cypress, frankincense, galbanum, geranium, lavender (English and spike), petitgrain, rose otto, tea tree

CHAKRA	LOCATION	ASSOCIATED PHYSIOLOGICAL SYSTEM	PSYCHO-SPIRITUAL/EMOTIONAL ATTRIBUTES	COLOR	ASSOCIATED GEMSTONES	ASSOCIATED SERENITY ESSENTIAL OILS
(4) Heart (Anahata)	Center of the chest	Circulatory	Balance, compassion, emotions, empathy, enthusiasm, ability to be gentle but firm, ideas, patience, self-determination and individuality, self-love, tolerance and acceptance of others, understanding	Green; also pink	Aventurine and rose quartz; also moss agate, apophyllite (green), chrysoprase, emerald, jade, malachite, rhodochrosite, tourmaline (green)	Mandarin (green) and rose otto; also cajeput, chamomile (German and Roman), cypress, frankincense, galbanum, geranium, lavender, spikenard, tea tree
(5) Throat (Vishuddha)	Just above the clavicle at the throat	Respiratory	Light blue range: dynamism, endocrine system balance, foresightedness, light-heartedness and happiness, persistence and success, spiritual growth, uprightness, ability to be goal oriented; Dark blue range: ability to face the truth, communication, connection between the inner self and the outside world, ability to convey feelings and emotions (to have our "voice"), dignity and honesty, personal inner truth, self-awareness, self-expression, sounds, verbal expression, wisdom	Blue	Aquamarine and lapis lazuli; also celestite, kyanite, topaz (blue), turquoise	Chamomile (German and Roman); also lavender (English and spike), spikenard

THE CHAKRAS: CONNECTIONS AND ASSOCIATIONS (continued)

CHAKRA	LOCATION	ASSOCIATED PHYSIOLOGICAL SYSTEM	PSYCHO-SPIRITUAL/EMOTIONAL ATTRIBUTES	COLOR	ASSOCIATED GEMSTONES	ASSOCIATED SERENITY ESSENTIAL OILS
(6) Third Eye (Ajna)	Between the eyebrows	Autonomic nervous system	Ability to face all experiences, concentration and higher thinking, insight, inspiration, intuition, psychic awareness self-knowledge, sense of justice, honesty and uprightness, vision (including inner vision)	Violet/ Purple	Amethyst; also azurite, iolite, lapis lazuli, rock crystal, sodalite, tanzanite	Patchouli; also frankincense, lavender (English and spike)
(7) Crown (Sahasrara)	The top of the head (crown)	Central nervous system	Higher awareness and consciousness, inspiration, harmonization of the nervous system, connection between spiritual self and physical self (channels vital energy to all chakras), imagination, positive thoughts, vitality of upper brain functions	Violet	Sugilite; also amethyst, apophylite, fluorite (purple)	Frankincense

Notes: I associate both green and pink with the heart chakra (4) to represent both pyscho-emotional and physiological qualities of the literal and metaphorical heart.

I use two primary gemstones with the throat chakra (5): aquamarine (light blue, leaning toward green) and lapis lazuli (dark blue, leaning toward indigo), depending on the intention behind the application.

All Serenity Essential Oils work on the third eye chakra (6) and the crown chakra (7) to varying degrees due to their psycho-emotional and spiritual influence; the ones listed in this chart are those that are especially influential.

ENERGY: YIN AND YANG

The ancient Chinese system of healing was (and continues to be) underpinned by the philosophical principle of primordial energy that manifests as two opposing yet complementary, polarized energetic forces. These forces—yin and yang—resonate in a perpetual state of flux that gives form and substance to the material and ethereal universe. When in perfect balance, or harmony, yin and yang are symbolically represented as two equal, interlinking halves of a whole circle, each perceivable by virtue of the contrasting or complementary existence of the other. Although one may predominate over the other (as one increases, the other decreases), dominance by either is never complete or constant—there always exists an element of yang in yin, and yin in yang. A shadow, for example, does not exist without light. Time is comprehensible because of the rhythm of day and night, the changing qualities of the seasons, the waxing and waning of the moon—there is constant, rhythmic, purposeful motion, change, and flux in the dynamic presence of yin and yang. Yin is represented by the dark (black) half of the symbolic circle and denotes qualities of femaleness, passivity, absorption, earth, darkness, night, and cold. Yang is represented by the light (white) half of the circle and denotes qualities of maleness, activity, penetration, heaven, light, day, and warmth.

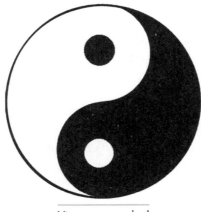

Yin-yang symbol

Examples of Opposing yet Complementary Qualities
Attributed to Yin and Yang

YIN	YANG
Earth	Heaven
Female	Male
Dark	Light
Passive/stasis	Active/movement
Absorption	Penetration
Night	Day
Moon	Sun
Cold	Warm
Negative	Positive
Solid	Hollow
Soft	Hard
Moisture	Dryness
Descending	Ascending
Contraction	Expansion
Intuitive	Logic
Liver	Gallbladder
Heart	Small intestine
Spleen-pancreas	Stomach
Lungs	Large intestine
Kidney	Urinary bladder
Essence (*jing*)	Mind (*shen*)
Blood and body fluids	Qi (chi)
Nutritive qi/chi	Defensive qi/chi
Breath in	Breath out
Even numbers	Odd numbers
Valleys	Mountains
Streams	Waterfalls
Tiger	Dragon
Orange	Azure
Black	White
- - - - - - (broken line)	_____ (solid line)

Essential oils possess both yin and yang qualities. Whether an oil is more yin than yang depends on various factors, which are not absolute. The plant requires soil (yang) and water (yin) to germinate. Roots (yang) reach down and spread into the earth (yin), and shoots (yin) push up through the earth toward sunlight (yang). Stems, tree trunks, buds, and fruits tend toward yin, while leaves, blossoms, and flowers tend toward yang. However, whether an essential oil is extracted from a root or a blossom does not mean it will exhibit the same tendencies; separated from the plant, the essential oil becomes an entity unto itself. Also, the chemical and energetic qualities of an essential oil alter from the moment of extraction and over time; the period of time allocated to distillation and the age and storage conditions of the essential oil, among other things, are determinant factors.

In the box below, I have characterized the Serenity Essential Oils based on my personal experience working with them. You will notice that based on their primary actions, some oils listed exhibit both yin and yang qualities, while others tend toward one or the other.

Yin and Yang Serenity Essential Oils

YIN	YIN/YANG	YANG
Chamomile (German)	Cajeput	Carrot seed
Cypress	Chamomile (Roman)	Frankincense
Geranium	Lavender (English and spike)	Galbanum
Petitgrain		Patchouli
Rose otto	Mandarin	Spikenard
Vetivert	Rose absolute	Tea tree

ELEMENTS

The philosophy of elemental energy originally developed as a secondary, parallel principle to that of yin and yang; both philosophies were later merged to depict and explain a complete, interactive system. The qualities of the five elements are symbolized by Wood, Earth, Water, Fire, and Metal. Each element represents a specific quality that complements and influences the movement and behavior of the others. These qualities manifest seamlessly within the body (mind-body-spirit) and environment (nature, the atmosphere, universe, and heavens). Essential oils balance and normalize these energetic qualities. They are physiologically and energetically protective and restorative. Their adaptogenic qualities promote dispersion of energetic excess and deficiency to restore natural flow between the elements. Again, you will notice below that the complex qualities of essential oils means their influence is often multidynamic.

YIN ELEMENTS	YIN/YANG ELEMENTS	YANG ELEMENTS
Water	Earth*	Fire
Metal		Wood

*According to Taoist philosophy, Earth can exist in either the yin or yang state and thus represents balance and unity. Earth contains the other four elements; its motion is inward and centering.

Serenity Essential Oils and the Five Elements

WATER	WOOD	FIRE	EARTH	METAL
Cajeput	Chamomile	Frankincense	Carrot seed	Cajeput
Chamomile	(Roman)	Mandarin	Galbanum	Chamomile
(German and	Lavender	Patchouli	Patchouli	(German)
Roman)	(English and	Petitgrain	Vetivert	Cypress
Cypress	spike)	Rose absolute		Frankincense
Geranium	Spikenard	Spikenard		Geranium
Rose otto				Lavender
Vetivert				(English and spike)
				Rose otto
				Tea tree

SERENITY ESSENTIAL OILS AND SUBTLE CONNECTIONS:
A QUICK REFERENCE GUIDE

ESSENTIAL OIL	COLOR(S)	GEMSTONE(S)	CHAKRA(S)	ELEMENT(S)	ENERGY
Cajeput	Green (also pink)	Aventurine (also rose quartz)	Heart	Metal, Water	Yin/yang
Galbanum	Yellow	Citrine	Solar plexus	Earth	Yang
	Green (also pink)	Aventurine (also rose quartz)	Heart		
Mandarin, green	Green (also pink)	Aventurine (also rose quartz)	Heart	Fire	Yin/yang
Petitgrain	Yellow	Citrine	Solar plexus	Fire	Yin
Tea tree	Yellow	Citrine	Solar plexus	Metal	Yang
	Green (also pink)	Aventurine (also rose quartz)	Heart		
Carrot seed	Orange	Carnelian	Sacral	Earth	Yang
	Yellow	Citrine	Solar plexus		
Chamomile, German	Green (also pink)	Aventurine (also rose quartz)	Heart	Metal, Water	Yin
	Blue	Aquamarine/ lapis lazuli	Throat		
Chamomile, Roman	Yellow	Citrine	Solar plexus	Water, Wood	Yin/yang
	Green (also pink)	Aventurine (also rose quartz)	Heart		
	Blue	Aquamarine/ lapis lazuli	Throat		
Cypress	Yellow	Citrine	Solar plexus	Water, Metal	Yin
	Green (also pink)	Aventurine (also rose quartz)	Heart		
Geranium	Yellow	Citrine	Solar plexus	Water, Metal	Yin

SERENITY ESSENTIAL OILS AND SUBTLE CONNECTIONS:
A QUICK REFERENCE GUIDE (continued)

ESSENTIAL OIL	COLOR(S)	GEMSTONE(S)	CHAKRA(S)	ELEMENT(S)	ENERGY
Geranium (continued)	Green (also pink)	Aventurine (also rose quartz)	Heart		
Lavender, English and spike	Yellow	Citrine	Solar plexus	Metal, Wood	Yin/yang
	Green (also pink)	Aventurine (also rose quartz)	Heart		
	Blue	Aquamarine/ lapis lazuli	Throat		
	Violet/ purple	Amethyst	Third eye		
	Violet	Sugilite	Crown		
Frankincense	Yellow	Citrine	Solar plexus	Fire, Metal	Yang
	Green (also pink)	Aventurine (also rose quartz)	Heart		
	Violet	Sugilite	Crown		
Patchouli	Orange	Carnelian	Sacral	Fire, Earth	Yang
	Violet/ purple	Amethyst	Third eye		
Rose otto	Yellow	Citrine	Solar plexus	Water, Metal	Yin
	Green (also pink)	Aventurine (also rose quartz)	Heart		
Rose absolute	Red	Jasper	Base	Fire	Yin/yang
	Orange	Carnelian	Sacral		
	Green (also pink)	Aventurine (also rose quartz)	Heart		
Spikenard	Red	Jasper	Root	Fire, Wood	Yang
	Orange	Carnelian	Sacral		
	Green (also pink)	Aventurine (also rose quartz)	Heart		
	Blue	Aquamarine/ lapis lazuli	Throat		
Vetivert	Red	Jasper	Root	Earth, Water	Yin
	Orange	Carnelian	Sacral		

6

Profiles

*Properties and Characteristics
of the Serenity Essential Oils*

The essential oils grouped together in the following two reference charts for addressing specific conditions share certain qualities with each other but also express their own unique profiles, or personalities. The recommended essential oils listed are a guide; find out more about the qualities of each one to ascertain its best match to you and your symptom expression. Each person will experience or express a condition or symptom in his or her own way and often for different reasons.

Please also note that, in the context of the information presented here, the terms *depression, anxiety, mood swings,* and the like refer to natural temporary psycho-emotional responses and fluctuations of mood and emotion provoked by day-to-day life events and circumstances. If your experience of any of these states is prolonged (over months) or occurs without obvious reason, you are advised to seek professional clinical diagnosis to eliminate other potential causes. Hypoglycemia, hyperventilation, food and chemical sensitivities and allergies, and withdrawal from medication or recreational drugs can also instigate feelings of anxiety and depression.

Before applying any of these oils to address the conditions cited, refer to the individual essential oil profiles in this chapter for further information. For a list of common skin conditions that can be treated with Serenity Essential Oils, including acne, eczema, psoriasis, dry skin, and burns, see pages 68–69.

Remember: Do not ingest essential oils. Oral ingestion of essential oils is *not* recommended unless under strict professional medical, and/or pharmaceutical or herbal guidance.

SERENITY ESSENTIAL OILS FOR COMMON PHYSIOLOGICAL CONDITIONS: A QUICK REFERENCE GUIDE

CONDITION	RECOMMENDED ESSENTIAL OILS	NOTES
Allergies	Chamomile (German and Roman), lavender (English)	These essential oils can relieve the symptoms of allergies; for true relief, the causes will need to be addressed.
Arthritis	Cajeput, carrot seed, chamomile (German and Roman), cypress, galbanum, lavender (spike), mandarin, petitgrain, vetivert	
Asthma	Chamomile (Roman), cypress, frankincense, galbanum, lavender (English), mandarin, petitgrain	Do not use essential oils at all during an asthma attack. Do not inhale essential oils if you are asthmatic; use only in a topical ointment, oil, or cream as a chest rub at a low dose (0.5 to 1% dilution). As a precaution, avoid rose essential oil; it may cause bronchospasm (Tisserand and Young 2014, 106).
Blood pressure, high or low	To regulate blood pressure: cypress, lavender (English), mandarin, rose otto	Massage regulates blood pressure. There is no evidence that essential oils can raise or lower blood pressure, but they may support the body's self-regulating processes. As a precaution, if you are taking medication for high blood pressure, avoid cypress essential oil.
Colds and flu	Cajeput, chamomile (German), cypress, frankincense, galbanum, geranium, lavender (English and spike), mandarin, petitgrain, tea tree	

CONDITION	RECOMMENDED ESSENTIAL OILS	NOTES
Drug addiction/ withdrawal	Spikenard, vetivert	These oils alleviate symptoms of withdrawal; they are calming and sedating. Drug withdrawal requires medical supervision.
Fungal infections	Cajeput, geranium, lavender (spike), patchouli, petitgrain, tea tree, vetivert	See pages 72–74 for more specific recommendations.
Headaches, migraine	Chamomile (German), spikenard, lavender (English and spike), rose otto	Inhalation of essential oils can cause a migraine; avoid direct inhalation during a migraine episode and use them topically instead (Tisserand and Young 2014, 105–9). A dab of neat lavender essential oil at each temple is often supportive for stress-related headaches.
Hyperactivity	Chamomile (Roman), frankincense, mandarin, petitgrain, spikenard, vetivert	
IBS (irritable bowel syndrome)	Carrot seed, lavender	Apply topically to the abdomen and lower back in a cream, vegetable oil, et cetera.
Joint pain	Cajeput, carrot seed, chamomile (German and Roman), cypress, galbanum, lavender (spike), mandarin, petitgrain	
Menstruation, painful	Chamomile (German and Roman), cypress, galbanum, geranium, lavender (spike), rose otto	Apply these essential oils topically, in a cream, oil, et cetera, to the abdomen and lower back before and during menstruation. Note that cypress may encourage bleeding and is best restricted to use before menstruation.
Myalgic encephalomyelitis/ chronic fatigue syndrome	Carrot seed, frankincense, geranium, lavender (English and spike), mandarin, petitgrain, rose otto (*Rosa × damascena*), tea tree, vetivert	These essential oils are all immune stimulants.
Muscles, aching	Chamomile (German and Roman), cypress, galbanum, lavender (English and spike), vetivert	

SERENITY ESSENTIAL OILS FOR
COMMON PHYSIOLOGICAL CONDITIONS:
A QUICK REFERENCE GUIDE (continued)

CONDITION	RECOMMENDED ESSENTIAL OILS	NOTES
PMS/menopause	Chamomile (German and Roman), cypress, frankincense, geranium, lavender (English), mandarin, patchouli, petitgrain, rose otto, spikenard, vetivert	
Stress and stress-related conditions	Carrot seed, chamomile (German and Roman), cypress, galbanum, geranium, frankincense, lavender (English), patchouli, petitgrain, rose, spikenard, vetivert	All Serenity Essential Oils support the body in stress management. The ones listed here are particularly effective.

SERENITY ESSENTIAL OILS FOR COMMON
PSYCHO-EMOTIONAL STATES:
A QUICK REFERENCE GUIDE

PSYCHO-EMOTIONAL STATE	SERENITY ESSENTIAL OIL
Agitation	Chamomile (German and Roman), lavender (English), rose otto
Anger	Chamomile (German and Roman), cypress, frankincense, geranium, petitgrain, rose otto
Anxiety	*Relaxing:* carrot seed, chamomile (German and Roman), cypress, frankincense, geranium, lavender (English), mandarin, petitgrain, rose otto, spikenard, vetivert *Stimulating (uplifting):* galbanum, geranium, patchouli, rose otto
Apathy	Cajeput, patchouli, tea tree
Confusion and indecisiveness	Carrot seed, cypress, frankincense, patchouli, vetivert
Depression and low mood	All Serenity Essential Oils, but especially chamomile (German and Roman), frankincense, galbanum, geranium, lavender (English and spike), mandarin, patchouli, petitgrain, rose otto, vetivert

PSYCHO-EMOTIONAL STATE	SERENITY ESSENTIAL OIL
Dwelling on unpleasant events	Cypress, frankincense
Fear and paranoia	Cypress, frankincense, rose otto
Grief	Cypress, frankincense, lavender (English), rose otto, spikenard
Hatred	Rose otto, spikenard
Hopelessness	Lavender (English and spike), petitgrain
Hypersensitivity	Chamomile (German and Roman), rose otto, vetivert
Impatience	Chamomile (German and Roman), cypress, lavender (English), frankincense, spikenard, vetivert
Inability to move on	Carrot seed, cypress, frankincense
Insomnia	Chamomile (German and Roman), frankincense, geranium (low dose), lavender (English) (low dose), mandarin, patchouli (low dose), rose otto (low dose), spikenard, vetivert
Irritability and intolerance	Chamomile (German and Roman), cypress, frankincense, lavender (English), spikenard
Jealousy	Geranium, rose otto
Mood swings	Geranium, lavender (English and spike), rose otto
Nervous tension	Chamomile (German and Roman), cypress, galbanum, geranium, lavender (English), mandarin, petitgrain, patchouli, spikenard, rose otto
Panic attacks	Chamomile (Roman), frankincense, lavender (English), patchouli, spikenard, vetivert
Resentment and disappointment	Frankincense, rose otto
Sadness and despair	Frankincense, rose otto
Shock	Lavender (English), rose otto, tea tree
Suspiciousness	Cypress, lavender (English)

Please note that the chemical constituents listed for each essential oil in the profiles that follow provides only a general overview. The exact composition of each individual essential oil will differ according to numerous contributing factors as described in chapter 2. Geographical location, altitude of growth, soil conditions, and so on will influence the chemical profile so that essential oils from the same botanical family or species will vary in composition.

German and Roman chamomile produce essential oils that are quite different in appearance, and I present their profiles separately, particularly for ease of application when using these oils with color and gemstones (as described in the previous chapter). In all other instances, the generic essential oil and closely related species of that particular oil are presented together for ease of comparison and selection; for example, English lavender and spike lavender as well as rose otto and rose absolute.

The CAS number assigned to each essential oil is the unique number, or identification code, attributed to it by the Chemical Abstracts Services (CAS); this number should appear on safety data information accompanying an essential oil through the chain of supply, from distiller to retailer.

CAJEPUT
(Melaleuca cajuputi)

Geographical location: Native to Australia; also grows in China, Malaysia, Indonesia, the Philippines, Vietnam, Java, Southeast Asia, and North America. *M. quinquenervia,* a species of cajeput, was introduced to Florida as an ornamental tree and to control swamp erosion; now considered invasive.

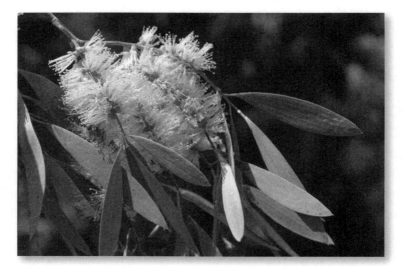

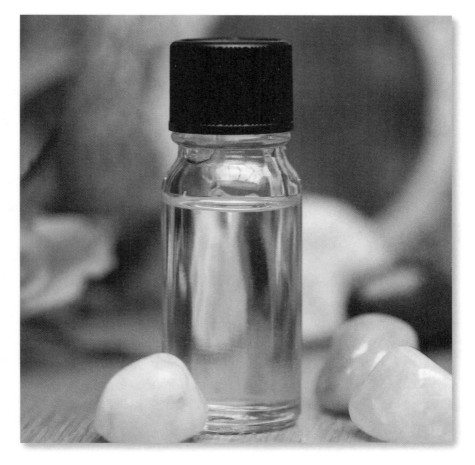

Plant description: An aromatic evergreen tree that grows to about 30 to 40 m high, with pale green oval leaves with pointed tips and white, cream, or greenish-yellow flowers carried on many-flowered spikes. The spongy flexible bark easily flakes from the trunk (and is used by Aborigines for shields, canoes, and roofing material). Also known as paperbark tree, punk tree, and white bottle brush tree. The name *cajeput* derives from the Indonesian *kayu putih*, "white wood."

Botanical family: Myrtaceae. Other species in the genus include *M. linariifolia, M. viridiflora,* and *M. symphocarpa.* Essential oils are extracted from *M. cajuputi* and *M. leucadendra.*

Extraction method: Steam distillation of the fresh leaves and twigs

Appearance of essential oil: Colorless to green, sometimes yellow

Odor of essential oil: Mild, sweet (fruity), fresh, camphoraceous, menthol, and metallic, with herbaceous greeny-woody notes; very faint herbaceous dry-out notes

Compatible Serenity Essential Oils for blending: Lavender (English and spike), petitgrain, rose otto

Safety data: Nontoxic, nonsensitizing. May be irritant to the skin and mucous membranes. Do not use during pregnancy or while breast-feeding. Poor-quality versions may be adulterated with eucalyptus, *M. quinquenervia,* or *M. symphyocarpa* essential oils and occasionally fixed oils or kerosene (Tisserand and Young 2014, 224). Assure authenticity/purity with your essential oil supplier.

Perfume Note: Top

Principal chemical constituents: CAS No.: 8008-98-8
1,8-cineole (41.1–70.8%), alpha-terpineol (6.5–8.7%), rho-cymene (0.7–6.8%), terpinolene (0.0–5.9%), gamma-terpinene (1.2–4.6%), (+)-limonene (3.8–4.1%), linalool (2.7–3.6%), alpha-pinene (2.1–3.2%), beta-caryophyllene (0.7–2.5%), beta-myrcene (0.9–2.0%), alpha-caryophyllene (0.5–1.6%), beta-pinene (0.8–1.5%), terpinen-4-ol (0.6–1.5%), alpha-selinene (0.0–1.5%), beta-selinene (0.0–1.5%), guaiol (0.0–1.2%)

(Tisserand and Young 2014, 223–24)

Subtle Connections

Color: Green *(opposite: red)*

Gemstone: Aventurine *(opposite: jasper)*

Chakra: Heart

Energy: Yin/yang

Element: Metal, Water

Actions and Uses

General actions: Analgesic, antiarthritic, antimicrobial, antiseptic, antispasmodic, bactericidal, expectorant

Skin: Acne, chapped and cracked skin, oily skin, pimples, psoriasis, insect bites

Respiratory system: Asthma, bronchitis, catarrhal infections, colds and flu, coughs, hay fever, laryngitis, sinusitis, sore throat, upper respiratory tract infections and pain

Joints and muscles: Arthritis, pain

Circulatory system: Varicose veins; supports venous and arterial tissue

Fungal infections: *Trichophyton* species (ringworm, athlete's foot, et cetera; see also page 74)

Associated limbic structure: Anterior thalamic nuclei

Potential psycho-emotional and spiritual support: Aids concentration, clears and stimulates the mind and thoughts, eases apathy, fosters courage in finding new pathways and managing change, strengthens resolve and spirit

CARROT SEED
(Daucus carota)

Geographical location: Originally native to Asia, then Europe, north Africa (Morocco, Algeria, Tunisia), and tropical Africa (Eritrea, Ethiopia) and naturalized in North America and Australia. The essential oil is produced mainly in France.

Plant description: Herbaceous annual (cultivated) or biennial (wild). Has a small inedible tough whitish root (cultivated species have fleshy orange taproots) with a stiff hairy stem. Grows up to 1 m high. Leaves are tripinnate, finely divided, and lacy. Flowers are small and

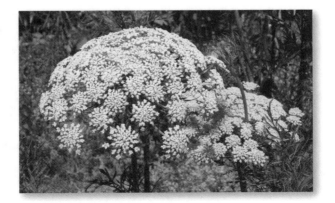

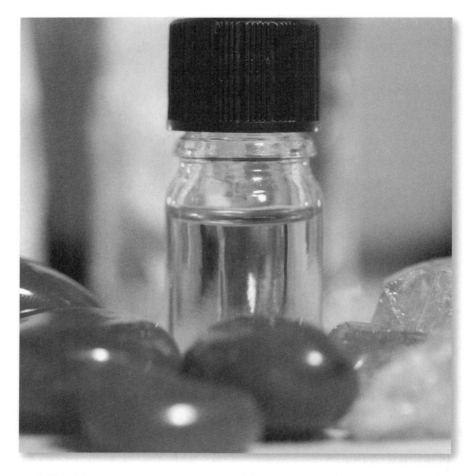

dull white, appearing in clusters of flat dense umbels; sometimes the flowers are pink in bud and reddish at the center of the umbel. The seeds, or fruits, are flat and green. The wild plant looks very similar to the deadly poisonous hemlock! Also known as wild carrot or Queen Anne's lace. (Domestic carrots are produced from cultivars of the subspecies *Daucus carota* subsp. *sativus*).

Botanical family: Umbelliferae

Extraction method: Steam distillation of the dried fruit (seeds)

Appearance of essential oil: Yellow to golden amber

Odor of essential oil: Dry, "carroty," slightly sweet, woody, earthy, mushroomy, and slightly herbaceous; slightly earthy, "carroty," and peppery at dry out

Compatible Serenity Essential Oils for blending: Geranium, lavender, mandarin

Safety data: Nontoxic, nonsensitizing, nonirritating. Avoid during pregnancy and while breastfeeding.

Perfume note: Middle

Principal chemical constituents: CAS No.: 8015-88-1

Carotol (36.1–73.1%), alpha-pinene (0.9–11.2%), daucene (1.6–5.9%), beta-caryophyllene (0.7–5.6%), (E)-dauc-8-en-4beta-ol (1.7–4.1%), sabinene (0.0–3.9%), geranyl acetate (0.0–3.7%), beta-bisabolene (1.5–3.1%), caryophyllene oxide (0.3–2.8%), (E)-beta-farnesene (1.6–2.5%), geraniol (0.0–2.2%), (E)-alpha-bergamotene (0.9–1.9%), daucol (1.2–1.7%), (–)-limonene (0.4–1.5%), beta-pinene (0.3–1.5%), beta-myrcene (0.4–1.3%), beta-selinene (0.0–1.1%), (Z)-alpha-bergamotene (0.0–1.1%)

(Tisserand and Young 2014, 233)

Subtle Connections

Colors: Orange *(opposite: blue),* yellow *(opposite: violet)*

Gemstones: Carnelian *(opposite: aquamarine/lapis lazuli),* citrine *(opposite: amethyst)*

Chakras: Sacral, solar plexus

Energy: Yang

Element: Earth

Actions and Uses

General actions: Antiarthritic, anti-infectious, anti-inflammatory, anti-oxidant (on the skin), smooth muscle relaxant, tonic

Skin: Abscesses, acne, chapped and cracked skin, dermatitis, dry skin, eczema, mature skin, psoriasis; detoxifies; revitalizes and improves the appearance of skin and scar tissue

Respiratory system: Chronic pulmonary conditions, bronchitis, coughs; strengthens mucous membranes

Joints and muscles: Accumulation of toxins, arthritis

Immune system: Chronic fatigue syndrome, myalgic encephalomyelitis

Digestive system: Colic, indigestion (with external application: inhalation, compress, ointment, or cream), irritable bowel syndrome

Associated limbic structures: Anterior thalamic nuclei, hypothalamus

Potential psycho-emotional and spiritual support: Eases anxiety, apathy, indecisiveness, mental and emotional exhaustion, and mental fog; calms experience of stress and confusion; helps with inability to move on; revitalizing; nervous system sedative

CHAMOMILE, GERMAN
(Matricaria recutita)

Geographical location: Native to Europe and temperate Asia and introduced to temperate North America and Australia. Grows wild near roads, around landfills, and in cultivated fields as a weed and

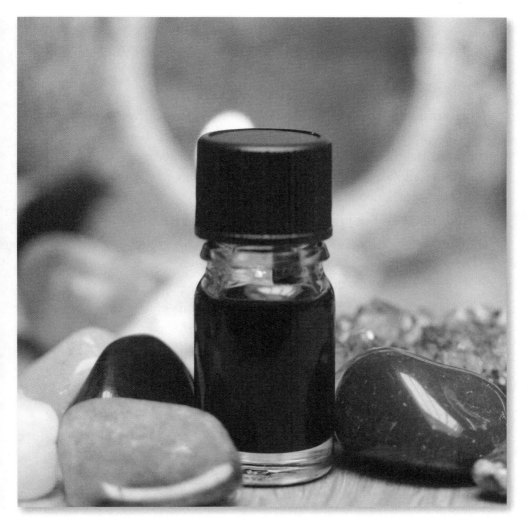

is also cultivated itself, particularly in Hungary and eastern Europe. Also known as blue chamomile, Hungarian chamomile, wild chamomile, false chamomile, or scented mayweed.

Plant description: A strongly aromatic annual herb growing up to 60 cm tall, with a smooth, erect, branching stem, delicate feathery fern-like leaves, and simple daisylike white flowers with a central yellow floret disk, presented on single stems. Similar in appearance to Roman chamomile, but the flower heads are smaller and have fewer petals. Under cultivation, the seeds are sown in spring or autumn and the flower heads are picked in full bloom in summer; this is an expensive and time-consuming operation as the staggered blooming of German chamomile flowers means that harvest has to be repeated over three to four weeks.

Botanical family: Asteraceae (Compositae)

Extraction method: Steam distillation of the flowering heads. Matricin, a sesquiterpene found in the plant, decomposes during this process to form the blue-colored compound chamazulene. An absolute is also produced in small quantities—it is deeper blue in color with greater tenacity and fixative properties.

Appearance of essential oil: Deep green-blue, turning to deep inky blue; moderately viscous

Odor of essential oil: Sweet, warm, herbaceous, fruity, haylike, with warm tobacco-like dry-out notes

Compatible Serenity Essential Oils for blending: Geranium, lavender, patchouli, rose otto

Safety data: Nontoxic, nonirritant; sensitizing only in rare cases . Prone to oxidization if not stored appropriately (in a cool, dark spot with a tightly secured lid). Poor-quality versions are sometimes adulterated with bisabolol and azulenes. Assure authenticity/purity with your essential oils supplier. Use in moderation. Possible CYP2C9, CYP1A2, and CYP34A enzyme interaction or drug substrate inhibition, although those interactions are seen mostly through oral ingestion (Tisserand and Young 2014, 58).

Perfume note: Middle

Principal chemical constituents: CAS No.: 8002-66-2 (farnesene/chamazulene chemotype*)

Farnesene (27.7%), chamazulene (17.6%), alpha-bisabolol oxide B (11.2%), alpha-bisabolol (9.6%), alpha-bisabolol oxide A (8.9%),

---

*There are various chemotypes of German chamomile, each identified by its predominant chemical: alpha-bisabolol, farnesene, or chamazulene. The content of alpha-bisabolol oxide (a sesquiterpene alcohol), for example, can range from 10 to 64 percent across the chemotypes. Bisabolol is not present in Roman chamomile. Bisabolol's predominant properties are anti-irritant, anti-inflammatory, and antimicrobial.

delta-cadinene (5.2%), alpha-muurolene (3.4%), (E)-beta-ocimene (1.7%), gamma-muurolene (1.3%)

(Tisserand and Young 2014, 242–43)

Subtle Connections

Colors: Green *(opposite: red),* blue *(opposite: orange)*

Chakras: Heart, throat

Gemstones: Aventurine *(opposite: jasper),* aquamarine/lapis lazuli *(opposite: carnelian)*

Energy: Yin

Elements: Metal, Water

Actions and Uses

General actions: Analgesic, antiallergenic, antiarthritic, anti-infectious, anti-inflammatory, antispasmodic, bactericidal, fungicidal (moderate), skin healing

Skin: Abscesses, acne rosacea, burns, chapped and cracked skin, dry/oily skin (balancing), infection, inflammation, psoriasis, puffiness, skin healing (very effective applied in low dosages)

Respiratory system: Asthma, catarrh, colds and flu, hay fever, mouth ulcers, teething, tonsillitis

Joints and muscles: Arthritis, inflamed joints, muscular aches and pains, neuralgia, rheumatism, sprains

Immune system: Immune support

Digestive system: Colic, indigestion, nausea (with external application: inhalation, compress, ointment, or cream)

Other: Headache, painful periods/PMS

Associated limbic structures: Anterior thalamic nuclei, hypothalamus

Potential psycho-emotional and spiritual support: Eases agitation, anxiety, depression/low mood, headaches, hypersensitivity, impatience, insomnia, irritability/intolerance, migraine, mood swings, nervous tension, and premenstrual tension; calms experience of stress; mental (calms an active mind) and nervous system sedative

CHAMOMILE, ROMAN
(Anthemis nobilis)

Geographical location: Native to southern and western Europe and naturalized in North America. Cultivated in England, Belgium, Hungary, Italy, France, North America, and Argentina. Flowers are harvested as they open in summer (June and July). Also known as English chamomile, garden chamomile, ground apple, low chamomile, or whig plant.

Plant description: Aromatic perennial flowering plant growing from 25 to 50 cm high, with feathery, finely dissected bipinnate leaves and solitary terminal white daisylike flowers with a prominent central yellow disk (the flowers are larger than those of German chamomile).

Botanical family: Asteraceae (Compositae)

Extraction method: Steam distillation of the flowering heads

Appearance of essential oil: Pale blue to straw yellow, or transparent to bluish-green

Odor of essential oil: Sweet, fruity (like ripe apple), and herbaceous, with warm, tealike dry-out notes

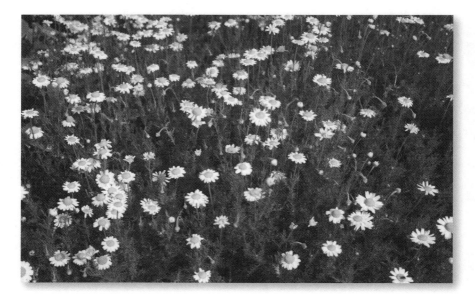

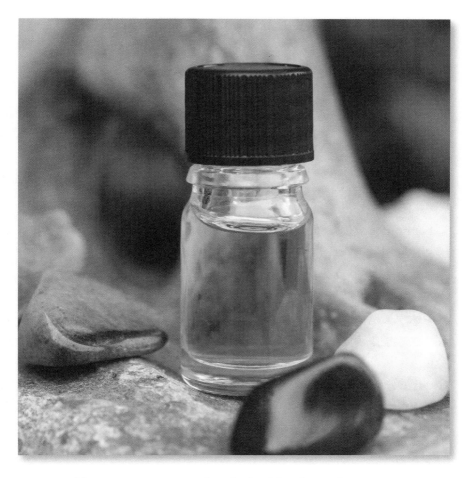

Compatible Serenity Essential Oils for blending: Cypress, geranium, lavender, rose otto

Safety data: Nontoxic, nonirritant, nonsensitizing. Prone to oxidization if not stored appropriately (in a cool, dark spot with a tightly secured lid). Poor-quality versions are sometimes adulterated with angelate, bisabolols, (Tisserand and Young 2014, 245; Burfeild 2003) or synthetic isobutyl angelate (Burfield 2003). Assure authenticity/purity with your essential oils supplier.

Perfume Note: Middle

Principal chemical constituents: CAS No.: 8015-92-7

Isobutyl angelate (0.0–37.4%), butyl angelate (0.0–34.9%), 3-methylpentyl angelate (0.0–22.7%), isobutyl butyrate (0.0–22.5%), isoamyl angelate (8.4–17.9%), 2-methyl-2-propenyl angelate (0.0–13.1%), 2-methyl-2-propyl angelate (0.0–7.4%), camphene (0.0–6.0%), borneol (0.0–5.0%), alpha-terpinene (0.0–5.5%), alpha-pinene (1.1–4.5%), chamazulene (0.0–4.4%), (E)-pinocarveol (0.0–4.4%), alpha-thujene (0.0–4.1%), hexyl butyrate (0.0–3.9%), terpinolene (0.0–3.9%), isobutyl isobutyrate (0.0–3.7%), anthemol (0.0–3.2%), gamma-terpinene (0.0–3.2%), isoamyl isobutyrate (0.0–3.1%), delta-3-carene (0.0–2.8%), isoamyl 2-methylbutyrate (0.0–2.8%), 2-methylbutyl 2-methylbutyrate (0.0–2.7%), isoamyl butyrate (0.0–2.6%), pinocarvone (0.0–2.4%), beta-myrcene (0.0–2.1%), rho-cymene (0.0–2.0%), beta-pinene (0.2–1.6%), isoamyl methacrylate (0.0–1.5%), beta-phellandrene (0.0–1.4%), propyl angelate (0.0–1.1%)

(Tisserand and Young 2014, 244–45)

Subtle Connections

Colors: Yellow *(opposite: violet)*, green *(opposite: red)*, blue *(opposite: orange)*

Gemstones: Citrine *(opposite: amethyst)*, aventurine *(opposite: jasper)*, aquamarine/lapis lazuli *(opposite: carnelian)*

Chakras: Solar plexus, heart, throat

Energy: Yin/yang

Elements: Water, Wood

Actions and Uses

General actions: Analgesic, antiarthritic, anti-infectious, antineuralgic, antiseptic, antispasmodic, bactericidal, nerve sedative, skin healing

Skin: Abscesses, acne, bruises, burns, chapped and cracked skin, dry/oily skin (balancing), eczema, dermatitis, itchy skin, psoriasis, puffiness, sensitive skin; skin healing; makes a good toner

Respiratory system: Asthma (especially nervous), mouth ulcers, teething

Joints and muscles: Arthritis, inflamed joints, muscular pain, neuralgia, sprains

Immune system: Immune support

Digestive system: Colic, indigestion (with external application: inhalation, compress, ointment, or cream), irritable bowel syndrome

Other: Painful periods/PMS

Associated limbic structures: Anterior thalamic nuclei, hypothalamus, amygdala

Potential psycho-emotional and spiritual support: Eases agitation, anger, anxiety, depression/low mood, fear, hyperactivity, hypersensivity, impatience, insomnia, irritability, panic attacks, premenstrual tension, restlessness, and solar plexus tension; calms experience of stress; mental, emotional, and nervous system sedative

CYPRESS
(Cupressus sempervirens)

Geographical location: Native to northern Persia, Syria, Turkey, Cyprus, and the Greek islands. Introduced to Europe by the Romans. Naturalized in eastern Mediterranean regions (it's known also as Mediterranean cypress), northeast Libya, southern Albania, Greece, Crete, Italy, northern Egypt, western Syria, Lebanon, Israel, Malta, Jordan, and Britain. Famous for its longevity (some trees are 1,000 years old). Also known as Italian cypress, Tuscan cypress, graveyard cypress, and pencil pine.

Plant description: Coniferous, statuesque evergreen tree growing up to 35 m tall. Dense dark-green foliage sprays, with tiny dark-green needlelike leaves. The small flowers produce oblong or ovoid seed cones (both male and female) that are initially green but turn brown when mature up to two years after pollination. Many cypress species produce essential oil; however, the *sempervirens* essential oil is considered to be of superior quality. The essential oil is produced mainly in France and Spain.

Botanical family: Cupressaceae

Extraction method: Steam distillation of the twigs and needles, and sometimes the cones

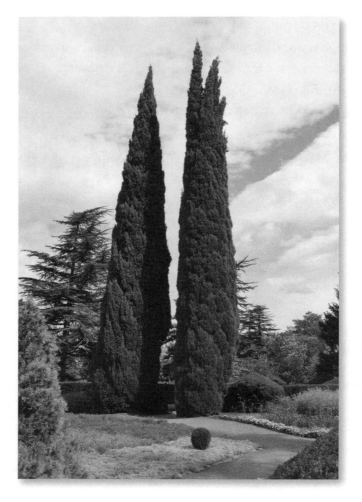

Appearance of essential oil: Colorless to green tinted, sometimes yellow tinted.

Odor of essential oil: Fresh, coniferous, and gently camphoraceous, with sweet and balsamic dry-out notes

Compatible Serenity Essential Oils for blending: Chamomile (Roman), lavender (English and spike), mandarin, spikenard

Safety data: Nontoxic, nonirritant, and nonsensitizing (although it can be sensitizing when oxidized, so be sure to include antioxidant ingredients, such as avocado oil, vitamin E oil, or carrot seed essential oil, to a cypress blend that you intend to store). Avoid during pregnancy (Tisserand and Young 2014, 265). Poor-quality versions

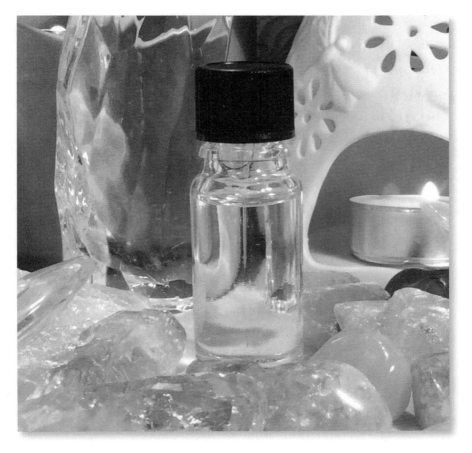

may be adulterated with synthetic alpha-pinene, delta-3-carene, and beta-myrcene (Burfield 2003). Assure authenticity/purity with your essential oils supplier.

Perfume note: Middle

Principal chemical constituents: CAS No.: 8013-86-3

Alpha-pinene (20.4–52.7%), delta-3-carene (15.2–21.5%), cedrol (2.0–7.0%), alpha-terpinyl acetate (4.1–6.4%), terpinolene (2.4–6.3%), (+)-limonene (2.3–6.0%), beta-pinene (0.8–2.9%), sabinene (0.7–2.8%), beta-myrcene (<2.7%), delta-cadinene (1.7–2.6%), terpinen-4-yl-acetate (1.2–2.1%), alpha-terpineol (1.2–1.4%), sandaracopimaradiene (0.2–1.3%), rho-cymene (0.2–1.2%), gamma-terpinene (0.4–1.1%), terpinen-4-ol (0.3–1.0%), borneol (trace–1.0%)

(Tisserand and Young 2014, 265)

Subtle Connections

Colors: Yellow *(opposite: violet)*, green *(opposite: red)*

Gemstones: Citrine *(opposite: amethyst)*, aventurine *(opposite: jasper)*

Chakras: Solar plexus, heart

Energy: Yin

Elements: Water, Metal

Actions and Uses

General actions: Antiarthritic, anti-infectious, anti-inflammatory, antiseptic, antispasmodic, astringent, antitussive (cough relieving), bactericidal, deodorant, mucolyptic

Skin: dry/oily skin (balancing), mature skin, perspiration (excessive), puffiness

Respiratory system: Asthma, bronchitis, colds and flu, dry throat, hoarseness, laryngitis, pulmonary infections, sinusitis, spasmodic cough, sore throat, upper respiratory tract infections and pain, whooping cough

Joints and muscles: Arthritis, muscular aches, pains, and cramps

Circulatory system: Blood pressure problems (helps the body with regulation, but do not use if taking medication), poor circulation

Immune system: Immune stimulant

Other: Painful periods/PMS (but note that cypress may encourage bleeding)

Associated limbic structures: Anterior thalamic nuclei, hypothalamus, amygdala, hippocampus

Potential psycho-emotional and spiritual support: Eases anger, anxiety, confusion and indecisiveness, fear/paranoia, grief, impatience, inability to concentrate, irritability, nervous tension, premenstrual tension, stress, stress-related conditions, and uncontrollable crying; helps with inability to move on or to stop dwelling on unpleasant events; regulates autonomic nervous system; sedative

FRANKINCENSE
(Boswellia carterii, B. sacra)

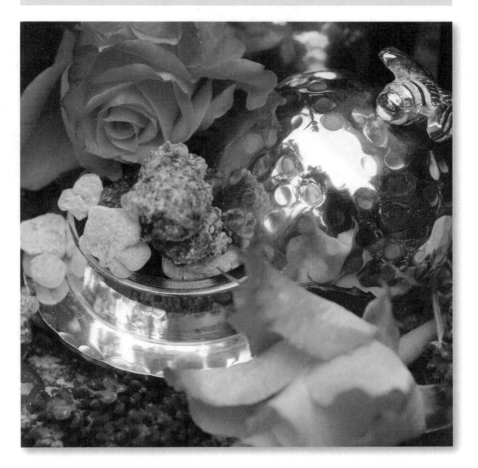

Geographical location: Native to the Red Sea region, growing in desert-woodland areas on rocky limestone slopes and gullies, particularly along the southern coastal mountains of the Arabian Peninsula, Somalia, Ethiopia, Southeast Asia, India, Sri Lanka, and China.

Plant description: The tree has a papery, peeling bark and tangled branches with abundant leaves. Oleo-gum-resin is extracted from the living tree by tapping the tree trunk via incisions made in the bark; the yellow, golden, or amber-brown exudates are left to dry and then removed. Distillation of the exudates takes place in Europe, Somalia,

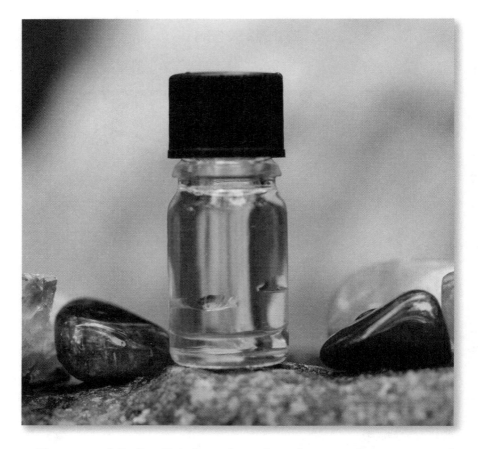

Yemen, and India. Dried exudates have been used as ceremonial incense in churches and temples and during indigenous rituals for thousands of years. The trees are endangered in some areas due to overharvesting of the resin (which reduces the reproductive capacity of the tree). Ensure that your essential oil supplier obtains their essential oil from a sustainable source.

Botanical family: Burseraceae. There are many frankincense species and chemotypes; in spite of this, from an ethnopharmacological perspective their properties are considered interchangeable. (This could have something to do with the fact that frankincense resin is often mixed with resin from other species or locations to manage profits and costs.) Resin from *Boswellia carterii* and *B. sacra* is believed to come from the same plant, although there is some dispute about this (Tisserand and Young 2014, 289).

Extraction method: Steam distillation of the dried oleo-gum-resin

Appearance of essential oil: Pale amber or yellow to greenish

Odor of essential oil: Fresh, lemony-fruity, green, and resinous. Slightly turpentine-like, woody middle notes with citrusy-sweet tones. Lingering woody, slightly citrusy, balsamic-herbaceous dry-out notes

Compatible Serenity Essential Oils for blending: Geranium, lavender (English and spike), mandarin, spikenard, vetivert

Safety data: Nontoxic, nonirritant, and nonsensitizing (although it can be sensitizing when oxidized, so be sure to include antioxidant ingredients, such as avocado oil, vitamin E oil, or carrot seed essential oil, to a frankincense blend that you intend to store). Some frankincense essential oils are derived from a mixture of resins or oils from various species (Tisserand and Young 2014, 288).

Perfume note: Base (to middle)

Principal chemical constituents: CAS No.: 8016-36-2 (alpha-pinene chemotype) (Middle East)

Alpha-pinene (10.3–51.3%), beta-phellandrene (0.0–41.8%), (+)-limonene (6.0–21.9%), beta-myrcene (0.0–20.7%), beta-pinene (0.0–9.0%), beta-caryophyllene (1.9–7.5%), rho-cymene (0.0–7.5%), terpinen-4-ol (0.0–6.9%), verbenone (0.0–6.5%), sabinene (0.0–5.5%), linalool (0.0–5.4%), alpha-thujene (0.0–4.5%), bornyl acetate (0.0–2.9%), delta-3-carene (0.0–2.6%), delta-cadinene (0.0–2.3%), camphene (0.0–2.0%), alpha-caryophyllene (0.0–1.8%), campholenic aldehyde (0.0–1.5%), octyl acetate (0.0–1.5%), caryophyllene oxide (0.0–1.4%), alpha-copaene (0.0–1.4%), calamenene (0.0–1.3%), thujol (0.0–1.2%), 1,8-cineole (0.0–1.0%), (E)-cinnamyl acetate (0.0–1.0%)

(Tisserand and Young 2014, 287–88)

Subtle Connections

Colors: Yellow *(opposite: violet)*, green *(opposite: red)*, violet *(opposite: yellow)*

Gemstones: Citrine *(opposite: amethyst)*, aventurine *(opposite: jasper)*, amethyst *(opposite: citrine)*

Chakras: Solar plexus, heart, crown

Energy: Yang

Elements: Fire, Metal

Actions and Uses

General actions: Anti-inflammatory, antiseptic, astringent, expectorant, skin healing, tonic

Skin: Burns, dermatitis, dry/oily skin (balancing), eczema, mature skin, scars, wound care

Respiratory system: Asthma, bronchitis, catarrh, colds and flu, coughs, shortness of breath, laryngitis, excessive mucus, sore throat, upper respiratory tract infections; calms breathing; encourages deep breathing

Circulatory system: Helps the body regulate blood pressure

Immune system: Chronic fatigue syndrome, myalgic encephalomyelitis; immune stimulant

Other: PMS, menopausal problems

Associated limbic structures: Anterior thalamic nuclei, hypothalamus, amygdala, hippocampus

Potential psycho-emotional and spiritual support: Eases anger, anxiety, confusion and indecisiveness, depression and low mood, fear and paranoia, grief, hyperactivity, impatience, irritability and intolerance, mood swings, nervous tension, panic attacks (calms and relaxes breathing), premenstrual tension, resentment and disappointment, and sadness and despair; helps with inability to move on, to stop dwelling on unpleasant events, or to let go of unwanted thoughts and memories; sedative; supports meditation and finding inner tranquillity

GALBANUM
(Ferula galbaniflua)

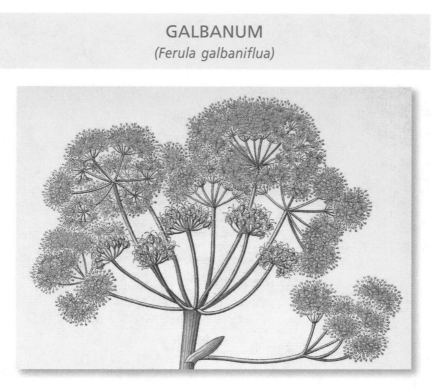

Geographical location: Native to the Middle East and western Asia; grows abundantly on the mountainous slopes in northern Iran; also cultivated in Afghanistan, Lebanon, and Turkey.

Plant description: Large perennial herb with a smooth hollow stem; shiny, finely toothed or serrated, pinnatifid, compound ovate leaflets; and umbels of small yellow flowers. The whole plant contains a milky white juice, produced in resinous ducts, that exudes from the base of the stem when it is cut down; incisions made in the harvested roots surrender most of this juice, which hardens into translucent-white, sometimes light-brown, yellowish, or greenish-yellow resinous "tears" or lumps. (The tears are sometimes waxy in texture—soft when warm, brittle when cold.) Distillation is undertaken in Europe and America.

Botanical family: Apiaceae (Umbelliferae)

Extraction method: Steam distillation of the oleo-gum-resin

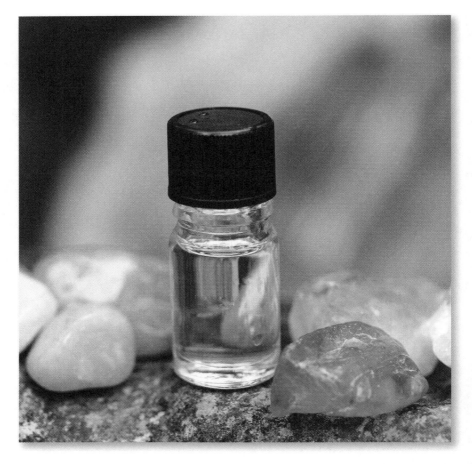

Appearance of essential oil: Clear to yellowish-brown or olive tinted

Odor of essential oil: Powerful, fresh, sharp, green, balsamic, slightly sweet, and herbaceous with earthy-woody undertones, finishing with dry, earthy, spicy dry-out notes

Compatible Serenity Essential Oils for blending: Geranium, lavender (English and spike)

Safety data: Nontoxic, nonirritant (when diluted, but potentially very irritating when undiluted), and nonsensitizing (although it can be sensitizing when oxidized, so be sure to include antioxidant ingredients, such as avocado oil, vitamin E oil, or carrot seed essential oil, to a galbanum blend that you intend to store) (Tisserand and Young 2014, 291).

Perfume note: Top

Principal chemical constituents: CAS No.: 8023-91-4

Beta-pinene (45.1–58.8%), alpha-pinene (5.7–12.0%), delta-3-carene (3.6–9.6%), sabinene (0.0–6.4%), beta-myrcene (0.0–4.6%), (+)-limonene (2.7–4.0%), gamma-elemene (0.0–2.4%), 1,3,5,-undecatriene (1.6–1.8%), (Z)-beta-ocimene (0.0–1.2%)

(Tisserand and Young 2014, 290–91)

Subtle Connections

Colors: Yellow *(opposite: violet)*, green *(opposite: red)*

Gemstones: Citrine *(opposite: amethyst)*, aventurine *(opposite: jasper)*

Chakras: Solar plexus, heart

Energy: Yang

Element: Earth

Actions and Uses

General actions: Analgesic, antiarthritic, anti-infectious, anti-inflammatory, antimicrobial, antispasmodic, astringent, decongestant, expectorant, restorative, skin healing

Skin: Abscesses, acne, boils, mature skin, pimples, psoriasis, scars; a good toner

Respiratory system: Asthma, bronchial spasms, catarrh, chronic coughs, colds and flu, mucous congestion

Joints and muscles: Arthritis, muscular pains; improves circulation

Other: Painful periods, menopausal symptoms

Associated limbic structure: Hypothalamus

Potential psycho-emotional and spiritual support: Balancing; both sedative and stimulant; calms erratic moods, nervous tension, menopausal symptoms, premenstrual tension, stress, and stress-related conditions; tonic; lifts mood and is restorative (nerves)

GERANIUM
(Pelargonium graveolens; Pelargonium × asperum)

Geographical location: Native to South Africa and widely cultivated in Russia, Egypt, Democratic Republic of the Congo, Japan, Central America, and Europe (Spain, Italy, and France).

Plant description: There are approximately 250 named species of *Pelargonium* (most are cultivated for ornamental purposes), but only *P. graveolens* and the very closely related *P. × asperum* are used for their essential oil. These are perennial hairy shrubs growing up to 1 m high, with serrated pointed leaves and small pink flowers. The whole plant is aromatic. Also known as rose geranium. The essential oil is mostly produced in China, Egypt, Morocco, Crimea, Ukraine, Georgia, India, Madagascar, and South Africa. *Pelargonium × asperum* is a cross between *P. capitatum* and *P. radens*.

Botanical family: Geraniaceae

Extraction method: Steam distillation of the leaves and stalks

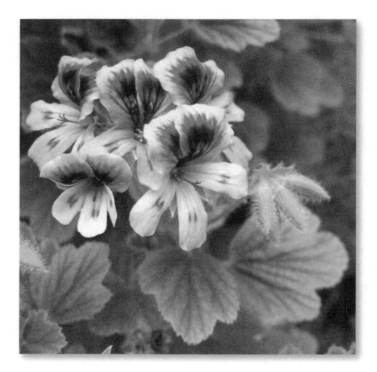

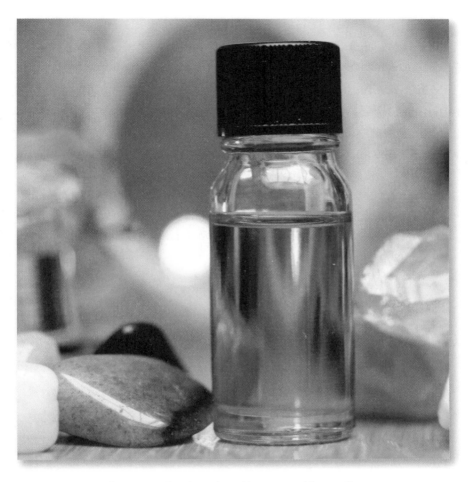

Appearance of essential oil: Pale yellow to golden yellow-green

Odor of essential oil: Rich, floral, roselike, sweet, and minty with a hint of lemon and greens, finishing with a green and roselike dry-out odor

Compatible Serenity Essential Oils for blending: Carrot seed, chamomile (Roman), frankincense, galbanum, lavender (English and spike), mandarin, petitgrain, rose otto, tea tree

Safety data: Nontoxic, nonirritant, and nonsensitizing (except in rare cases, and then more particularly with the highly perfumed Bourbon type, which is rarely found in the aromataherapy market; use in moderation as a caution). Indian geranium oil (which may contain diphenyl oxide—a synthesized chemical mixture with a geranium-like odor, used as an ingredient in perfumary) is sometimes added to Chinese geranium oil to improve profitability (Burfield 2003). Assure authenticity/purity with your essential oils supplier.

Perfume note: Middle

Principal chemical constituents: CAS No.: 8004-46-2 (Egyptian geranium)

Citronellol (24.8–27.7%), geraniol (15.7–18.0%), linalool (0.5–8.6%), citronellyl formate (6.5–6.7%), isomenthone (5.7–6.1%), 10-epi-gamma-eudesmol (5.5–5.7%), geranyl formate (3.6–3.7%), geranyl butyrate (1.5–1.9%), geranyl tiglate (1.5–1.9%), beta-caryophyllene (1.2–1.3%) germacrene D (0.3–1.2%), guaia-6,9-diene (0.3–1.2%), geranyl propionate (1.0–1.1%), (Z)-rose oxide (0.9–1.0%), 2-phenylethyl butyrate (0.0–1.0%)

(Tisserand and Young 2014, 292–94)

Subtle Connections

Colors: Yellow (*opposite: violet*), green (*opposite: red*)

Gemstones: Citrine (*opposite: amethyst*), aventurine (*opposite: jasper*)

Chakras: Solar plexus, heart

Energy: Yin

Elements: Water, Metal

Actions and Uses

General actions: Antibacterial, antifungal, anti-inflammatory, antiseptic, astringent, deodorant

Skin: Abscesses, acne, burns, bruises, chapped and cracked skin, dermatitis, dry/oily skin (balancing), eczema, herpes simplex, mature skin, shingles

Respiratory system: Asthma, colds and flu, infections, excessive mucus, sore throat, tonsillitis

Joints and muscles: Cellulitis, edema

Immune system: Chronic fatigue syndrome, myalgic encephalomyelitis, viral infections (including shingles); immune stimulant

Fungal infections: *Candida* species (ringworm, athlete's foot, et cetera; see page 72)

Other: Painful periods, PMS, menopausal problems

Associated limbic structures: Anterior thalamic nuclei, hypothalamus, amygdala, hippocampus

Potential psycho-emotional and spiritual support: Both sedative and stimulant; eases anxiety, depression and low mood, headaches, jealousy, nervous tension, menopausal symptoms, mood swings, premenstrual tension, stress, and stress-related conditions; balances the nerves and solar plexus; uplifting; endocrine stimulant (hormone-like)

LAVENDER—ENGLISH (Lavandula angustifolia) AND SPIKE (L. latifolia)

Geographical location: Native to the Mediterranean, particularly France and the Pyrenees mountains in northern Spain. Cultivated in England, Norway, Italy, Greece, Turkey, Bulgaria, the former Yugoslavia, Russia, Australia, and Tasmania.

Plant description: (English, *L. Angustifolia*) Woody evergreen, compact bushy shrub growing up to 1 m high, with narrow aromatic gray-green leaves and small tubular pale to deep purple flowers on dense blunt spikes. The whole plant is highly aromatic. Harvested toward the end of flowering and distilled when fresh.

(Spike, *L. latifolia*) Similar in appearance to *L. angustifolia* but with pale gray-blue flowers at the top of long single stemmed leafless spikes with broad gray-green leaves. Grows up to 80 cm high. Grows at a lower altitude and has a higher plant yeild than *L. angustifolia*.

Botanical family: Lamiaceae (Labiatae)

Extraction method: Steam distillation of the fresh flowering tops

Appearance of essential oil: Clear to pale yellow-green

Odor of essential oil: (English, *L. Angustifolia*) Fresh, floral, fruity to herbaceous, and slightly woody; nondescript at dry out. English

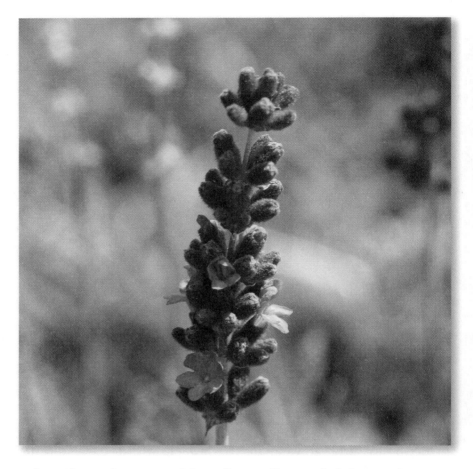

lavender is characterized by softer, mellower, slightly rounder notes compared to French lavenders and other lavender oils.

(Spike, *L. latifolia*) Fresh and strongly camphoraceous with herbaceous-woody dry-out notes (sometimes described as a cross between sage and lavender)

Compatible Serenity Essential Oils for blending: Cajeput, carrot seed, chamomile (German and Roman), cypress, frankincense, galbanum, geranium, mandarin, patchouli, spikenard, tea tree, vetivert

Safety data: Nontoxic, nonirritant, and nonsensitizing (though there is moderate risk of sensitization if it is overused). Spike lavender may be mildly neurotoxic due to its camphor content (Tisserand and Young 2014, 326–27, 329). English lavender may be adulterated with

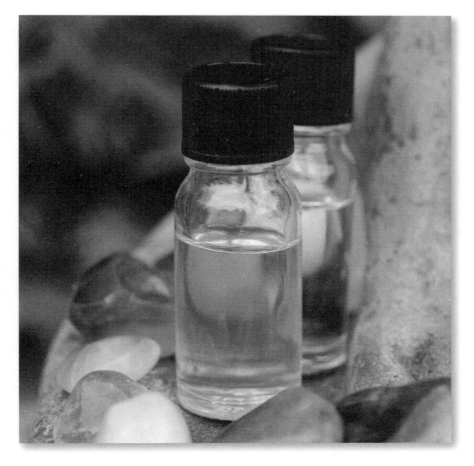

cheaper lavandin *(Lavandula × intermedia)* oil varieties, spike lavender essential oil, rectified ho oil *(Cinnamomum* spp.), acetylated ho or acetylated lavandin oils, et cetera (Burfield 2003). Assure authenticity/purity with your essential oils supplier.

Perfume note: Middle (to top)

Principal chemical constituents: CAS No.: 8000-28-0 (English)
Linalyl acetate (20.0–50.0%), linaool (20.0–50.0%), cis-beta-ocimene (1.0–5.0%), beta-caryophyllene (1.0–5.0%), trans-beta-ocimene (1.0–5.0%), 4-carvomenthenol (1.0–5.0%), alpha-terpineol (1.0–5.0%), l-limonene (0.1–1.0%), camphene (0.1–1.0%), beta-pinene (0.1–1.0%), geraniol (0.1–1.0%)

(Norfolk Essential Oils 2017)

CAS No.: 8016-78-2 (Spike)

Linalool (27.2–43.1%), 1,8-Cineole (28.0–34.9%), Camphor (10.9–23.2%), Borneol (0.9–3.6%), beta-pinene (0.8–2.6%), (E)-alpha-Bisabolene (0.5–2.3%), alpha-pinene (0.6–1.9%), beta-caryophyllene (0.5–1.9%), alpha-terpineol (0.8–1.6%), Germacrene D (0.3–1.0%)

(Tisserand and Young 2014, 329)

Subtle Connections

Colors: Yellow (*opposite: violet*), green (*opposite: red*), blue (*opposite: orange*), violet/purple (*opposite: yellow*)

Gemstones: Citrine (*opposite: amethyst*), aventurine (*opposite: jasper*), aquamarine/lapis lazuli (*opposite: carnelian*), amethyst (*opposite: citrine*)

Chakras: Solar plexus, heart, throat, third eye, crown

Energy: Yin/yang

Elements: Metal, Wood

Actions and Uses

General actions: Analgesic, antiarthritic, antidepressant, anti-infectious, anti-inflammatory, antimicrobial, antiseptic, antispasmodic, bactericidal, cleansing, deodorant, hypotensive, mucolytic, skin healing, tonic, toxin neutralizing

Skin: Abscesses (spike lavender), acne, bruises, burns, chapped and cracked skin, dry/oily skin (balancing), dermatitis, eczema, insect bites, itchy skin, mature skin, pimples, psoriasis, ringworm, shingles, scars

Respiratory system: *English lavender:* asthma, bronchitis, catarrh, colds and flu, gingivitis, halitosis, hay fever, laryngitis, panic attacks, pulmonary infections and viruses, sore throat, upper respiratory infections; *spike lavender:* asthma, bronchitis, hay fever, laryngitis, sinusitis, tonsillitis

Joints and muscles: Arthritis (spike lavender), muscle aches and pains, sciatica, sprains

Circulatory system: Helps the body regulate blood pressure

Immune system: Chronic fatigue syndrome, myalgic encephalomyelitis; immune stimulant (spike lavender); immune support (English lavender)

Fungal infections: *Malassezia* species (spike lavender; see page 73)

Other: Headaches, migraine, painful periods/PMS, menopausal problems

Associated limbic structures: Anterior thalamic nuclei, hypothalamus, amygdala

Potential psycho-emotional and spiritual support: Sedative at low dosages, stimulant at high dosages; eases agitation, anger, anxiety, depression, grief, headaches, insomnia, irritability, manic depression (professional support required), mood swings, nervous tension, panic, premenstrual tension, sense of hopelessness, shock, solar plexus tension, stress, stress-related conditions, and suspiciousness

MANDARIN, GREEN
(Citrus reticulata)

Geographical location: Native to southeastern Asia and the Philippines, especially southern China, Japan, and the East Indies. Introduced to Europe and then America (where it was renamed tangerine) in the 1800s. Now cultivated and produced mainly in Italy, Spain, Algeria, Cypress, Greece, the Middle East, Brazil, and the United States (Alabama, Florida, Mississippi, Texas, Georgia, and California). There are many cultivars. The names tangerine, satsuma, and mandarin are sometimes used interchangeably, even though each represents a different chemotype.

Plant description: Small evergreen, usually thorny tree growing up to 7.5 m high (mandarin trees are usually smaller than sweet orange trees, depending on the variety). The leaves are broad or slender, lanceolate, and glossy with minute rounded teeth, and the very fragrant flowers are single or clustered. The fleshy fruits are deep green, bright orange, or red-orange and have a loose peel. The tangerine is larger and rounder than the mandarin, with a yellowish skin,

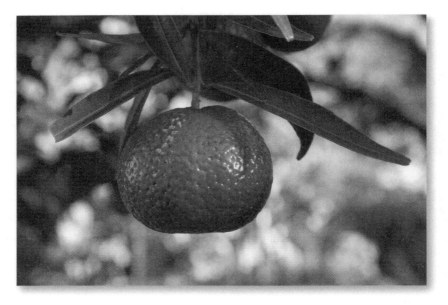

more like the original Chinese mandarin type. Also known as mandarin orange.

Botanical family: Rutaceae

Extraction method: Cold expression of the outer peel

Appearance of essential oil: Mid to dark olive green

Odor of essential oil: Initial but fleeting sharp notes, fresh, warm, fruity, intense, deep, sweet, and softly citrusy with obvious mandarin peel odor, fading to faintly fruity, tangeriney, soft, and fruity until it is barely detectable.

Compatible Serenity Essential Oils for blending: Carrot seed, cypress, geranium, frankincense, patchouli, petitgrain, tea tree

Safety data: Nontoxic, nonirritating, and generally nonsensitizing (although it can be sensitizing when oxidized, so be sure to include antioxidant ingredients, such as avocado oil, vitamin E oil, or carrot seed essential oil, to a mandarin blend that you intend to store) (Tisserand and Young 2014, 342).

Perfume note: Top

Principal chemical constituents: CAS No.: 8008-31-9

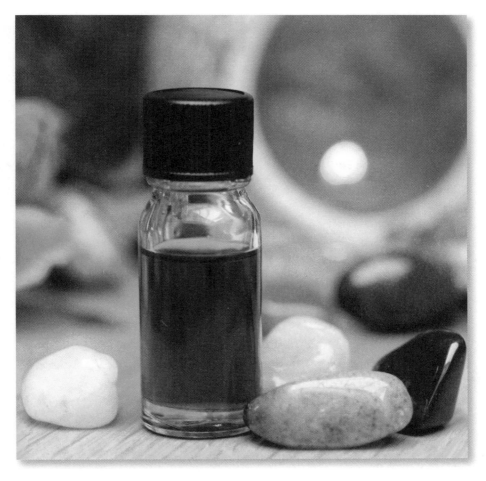

D-limonene (65.0–75%), gamma-terpinene (16.0–22.0%), alpha-pinene (2.0–4.0%), beta-pinene (1.5–3.0%), beta-myrcene (1.5–3.0%) (NHR Organic Oils 2015)

Subtle Connections

Color: Green *(opposite: red)*

Gemstone: Aventurine *(opposite: jasper)*

Chakra: Heart

Energy: Yin/yang

Element: Fire

Actions and Uses

General actions: Antiseptic, antispasmodic, bactericidal, cleansing, hydrating, skin healing, tonic for the skin and body

Skin: Acne, congested and oily skin, scars, spots, stretch marks

Respiratory system: Asthma, bronchitis, colds and flu, coughs

Joints and muscles: Arthritis, fluid retention

Circulatory system: Helps the body regulate blood pressure

Immune system: Chronic fatigue syndrome, myalgic encephalomyelitis; immune stimulant

Other: PMS, menopausal problems

Associated limbic structures: Hypothalamus, amygdala

Potential psycho-emotional and spiritual support: Awakens; brings out the inner child; good for quelling anxiety, depression and low mood, hyperactivity (although orange can encourage hyperactivity, mandarin is calming), insomnia, nervous tension, panic attacks, premenstrual tension, restlessness, stress, and stress-related conditions; has a sedative quality

PATCHOULI
(Pogostemon cablin)

Geographical location: Native to tropical regions of Asia and cultivated in China, Indonesia, India, Malaysia, Mauritius, Taiwan, the Philippines, Thailand, Vietnam, West Africa, and South America. The essential oil is mainly distilled in Europe and America from imported dried leaves.

Plant description: Perennial fragrant bushy herb growing up to 1 m high, with sturdy erect hairy square stems, large furry oval leaves, and spikes bearing small white or pale pink to light purple flowers. The shoots and leaves are harvested two or three times a year (the leaves are usually partially fermented before distillation).

Botanical family: Lamiaceae (Labiatae)

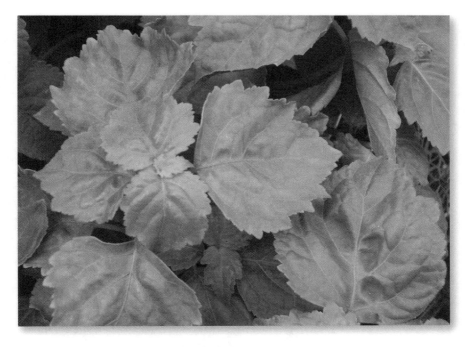

Extraction method: Steam distillation of the dried partially fermented leaves

Appearance of essential oil: Amber or dark orange to thick brown or yellowish-amber; viscous

Odor of essential oil: Sweet, rich, herbaceous, balsamic, earthy, and mossy-woody to slightly camphoraceous and spicy, finishing with a lingering, tenacious dry, woody balsamic-spicy dry-out odor

Compatible Serenity Essential Oils for blending: Geranium, lavender (English and spike), mandarin, rose otto, spikenard, vetivert

Safety data: Nontoxic, nonirritant, and nonsensitizing. Sometimes adulterated with gurjun balsam oil, copaiba balsam oil, cedarwood oil, distillate residue from patchouli, vetivert, and camphor, and vegetable oils, among others (Tisserand and Young 2014, 382). The superior Indonesian patchouli oil is often blended with the cheaper Chinese oil (Burfield 2003). Assure authenticity/purity with your essential oils supplier.

Perfume note: Base (to middle)

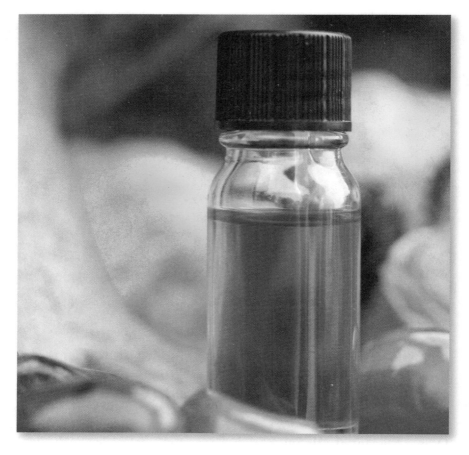

Principal chemical constituents: CAS No.: 8014-09-3 (Indonesian)
Patchoulol (28.2–32.7%), alpha-bulnesene/delta-guaiene (15.8–18.8%),
alpha-guaiene (13.5–14.6%), seychellene (0.0–9.0%), gamma-patchoulene
(0.0–6.7%), alpha-patchoulene (4.5--5.7%) beta-caryophyllene (3.1–4.2%),
1(10)-aromadendrene (0.0–3.7%), beta-patchoulene (2.0–3.4%), pogostol
(trace–2.4%), (–)-allo-aromadendrene (0.0–2.4%), delta-cadinene
(0.0–2.4%)

(Tisserand and Young 2014, 382)

Subtle Connections

Colors: Orange *(opposite: blue),* violet *(opposite: yellow)*

Gemstones: Carnelian *(opposite: aquamarine/lapis lazuli),* amethyst
(opposite: citrine)

Chakras: Sacral, third eye

Energy: Yang

Elements: Fire, Earth

Actions and Uses

General actions: Antidepressant, anti-infectious, anti-inflammatory, antimicrobial, antiseptic, antiviral, astringent, bactericidal, deodorant, fungicidal, skin healing, toxin neutralizing

Skin: Abscesses, chapped and cracked skin, dandruff, dermatitis, eczema, impetigo, insect bites (also an insect repellent), oily scalp and skin, scars, sores, wounds, wrinkles/mature skin

Respiratory system: Calms and regulates breathing

Immune system: Immune support

Fungal infections: *Candida* species (ringworm, athlete's foot, et cetera; see page 73)

Other: PMS, menopause; endocrine stimulant

Associated limbic structures: Anterior thalamic nuclei, hypothalamus, and pituitary (via the hypothalamus)

Potential psycho-emotional and spiritual support: Sedative at low dosages, stimulant at high dosages; eases apathy, confusion and indecisiveness, depression and low mood, nervous exhaustion, nervous tension, panic attacks, premenstrual tension, stress, and stress-related conditions; endocrine stimulant; supports meditation and a sense of spirituality

PETITGRAIN
(Citrus aurantium var. amara)

Geographical location: Native to southern China and northeastern India and cultivated in Paraguay, France, North Africa, and Haiti. France produces the best-quality petitgrain essential oil (which is used mainly as a perfume ingredient), although Paraguay also produces an intensely perfumed version. Known also as orange leaf oil or mandarin leaf oil.

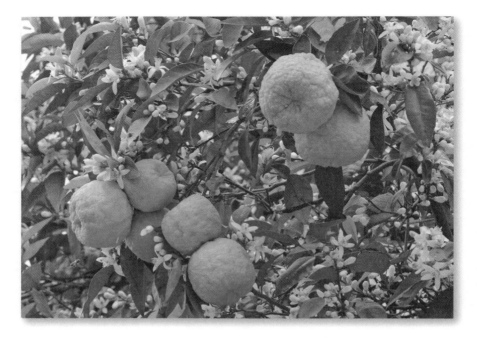

Plant description: An evergreen aromatic tree growing up to 10 m high (but only about 6 m high when growing wild) with a smooth brown trunk, stout branches, leathery dark green leaves, fragrant blossoms, and small bitter orange fruits. An essential oil is extracted from both the blossoms (neroli) and the fruits (bitter orange). Petitgrain essential oil is extracted from the leaves and twigs. A type of petitgrain is also produced from lemon, sweet orange, mandarin, and bergamot trees.

Botanical family: Rutaceae

Extraction method: Steam distillation of the leaves and twigs

Appearance of essential oil: Clear to pale yellow, yellow to amber

Odor of essential oil: Fresh and floral, woody, citrusy/orange-like; similar tones to neroli. Dry, floral, herbaceous, with dry and herbaceous dry-out notes

Compatible Serenity Essential Oils for blending: Geranium, lavender (English and spike), mandarin

Safety data: Nonirritant, nontoxic, and nonsensitizing. The more expensive petitgrain bigarade (petitgrain from the bitter orange tree)

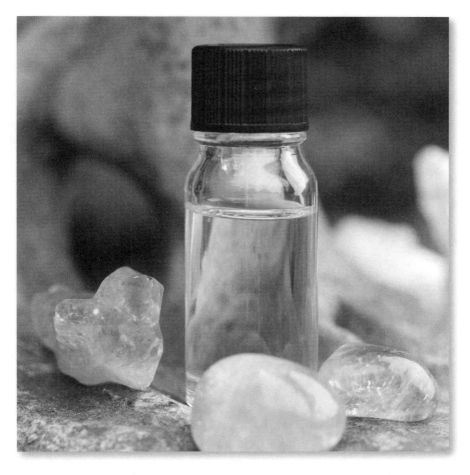

may be adulterated with cheaper Paraguayan petitgrain oil (Tisserand and Young 2014, 375). All petitgrain essential oils may be adulterated with the addition of other citrus leaf oils and fractions, fatty aldehydes, linalyl acetate, orange terpenes, and so on. Paraguayan oil is often adulterated with synthetic linalool, linalyl acetate, alphaterpineol, geranyl acetate, neryl acetate, trace amounts of pyrazines, among other things (Burfield 2003). Assure authenticity/purity with your essential oils supplier.

Perfume note: Top

Principal chemical constituents: CAS No.: 8016-44-2 (Paraguayan) Linalyl acetate (47.4–58.0%), linalool (20.8–25.2%), alpha-terpineol (4.4–6.8%), geranyl acetate (2.9–4.5%), geraniol (2.1–3.0%), neryl acetate (2.1–3.0%), beta-myrcene (0.0–2.0%), (E)-beta-ocimene (0.0–2.0%), beta-pinene (0.3–1.2%), (+)-limonene (0.3–1.1%)

CAS No.: 8014-17-3 (Bigarade)
Linalyl acetate (51–71%), linalool (12.3–24.2%), (+)-limonene (0.4–8.0%), alpha-terpineol (2.1–5.2%), geranyl acetate (1.9–3.4%), beta-pinene (0.3–2.7%), neryl acetate (0.0–2.6%), geraniol (1.4–2.3%), (E)-beta-ocimene (0.2–2.2%), beta-myrcene (0.0–2.0%), nerol (0.4–1.1%)

(Tisserand and Young 2014, 374–75)

Subtle Connections

Color: Yellow *(opposite: violet)*

Gemstone: Citrine *(opposite: amethyst)*

Chakra: Solar plexus

Energy: Fire

Element: Yin

Actions and Uses

General actions: Antiarthritic, anti-infectious, anti-inflammatory, antiseptic, antispasmodic, deodorant, tonic

Skin: Acne, chapped and cracked skin, dry/oily skin or scalp (balancing), perspiration (excessive), scars

Respiratory system: Asthma (nervous), colds and flu, hay fever, respiratory infections; eases breathing, including shallow breathing brought on by stress

Joints and muscles: Arthritis, joint inflammation

Immune system: Chronic fatigue syndrome, myalgic encephalomyelitis; immune stimulant

Fungal infections: *Candida* and *Microsporum* species (ringworm, athlete's foot, et cetera; see also page 73)

Other: PMS, menopausal problems

Associated limbic structures: Hypothalamus and amygdala

Potential psycho-emotional and spiritual support: Eases anger, anxiety, depression, hyperactivity, insomnia, mental fog, nervous exhaustion, nervous tension, premenstrual tension, sense of hopelessness, stress, and stress-related conditions; nervous system sedative

ROSE OTTO
(Rosa × damascena, Rosa × centifolia)

Geographical location: Originally native to eastern Asia and the Middle East. Japan, Morocco, Tunisia, and Iran have a historical association with rose dating back thousands of years; however, the largest producers of rose today are Bulgaria and Turkey, followed by France and India and, to a lesser degree, the Middle East. India specializes in producing rose otto (or rose attar, as it's also known), absolutes, and concretes. *Rosa × damascena* is strictly a cultivated species.

Plant description: *Rosa × damascena* (commonly known as damask rose or the rose of Castile) is a hybrid derived from *Rosa gallica* and *Rosa moschata,* originally cultivated hundreds of years ago. It is a deciduous, informally shaped shrub growing up to 2.2 m high with curved prickles and stiff bristles protruding from its stem, pinnate leaves, and relatively small pink to light red, highly fragrant, multipetaled flowers that grow in clusters.

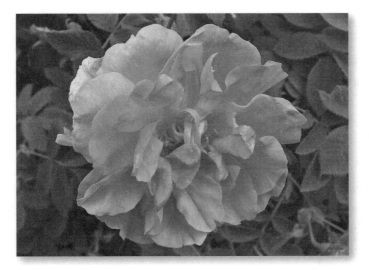

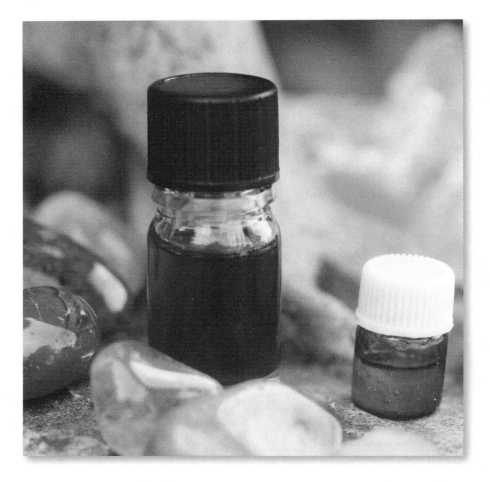

Rosa × *centifolia* (also known as Provence rose or cabbage rose), a derivative of *Rosa* × *damascena,* was originally cultivated in Holland between the seventeenth and nineteenth centuries. It is similar in stature to the damask rose, though slightly shorter, growing up to 2 m high, with long drooping cane-like stems, green-gray pinate leaves, and highly fragrant, multipetaled, globular pink, or sometimes white to dark red-purple, flowers.

Botanical family: Rosaceae

Extraction method: Water or steam distillation of the fresh petals; labor intensive to produce (flowers must be hand-picked), with a relatively low yield of essential oil per volume of plant material, rendering the oil very expensive

Appearance of essential oil: Pale yellow or olive (depending on the color of the petals from which it is distilled); the oil crystallizes (solidifies) at low temperatures

Appearance of absolute: Deep orange-red to olive green viscous liquid

Odor of essential oil: Powerful, complex, sweet, fresh, highly floral and beeswax-like, with a tenacious soft, warm, floral dry-out odor

Odor of absolute: Rich, intense, fresh, warm, deeply floral, almost intoxicating, with tenacious lingering floral-citrusy dry-out notes. The absolute is used extensively in perfumery.

Compatible Serenity Essential Oils for blending: Most Serenity Essential Oils, but especially chamomile (German and Roman), geranium, lavender (English and spike), patchouli, and vetivert

Safety data: Nonirritant, nontoxic, and non-sensitizing (but highly perfumed, so use it in low doses). Although it contains methyleugenol, which is considered potentially carcinogenic, evidence suggests that the presence of geraniol apparently counteracts the effect of this compound (Tisserand and Young 2014, 406). Rose absolute should be regarded like a perfume, having irritant and sensitizing potential. Poor-quality essential oils are often adulterated with synthetic reconstructions of various constituents, ethanol, 2-phenylethanol, fractions of geranium oil, and cheaper rose oils (Burfield 2003; Tisserand and Young 2014, 405). Assure authenticity/purity with your essential oils supplier.

Perfume note: Base (very tenacious) to middle (with intense but fleeting top notes)

Principal chemical constituents: CAS No.: 8007-01-0 (Damask, Bulgarian—otto)

(–)-Citronellol (16.0–35.9%), geraniol (15.7–25.7%), alkenes (such as gamma-muurolene, alpha-pinene) and alkanes (such as tricosane, eicosane, octadecane) (19.0–24.5%), nerol (3.7–8.7%), methyleugenol (0.5–3.3%), linalool (0.4–3.1%), citronellyl acetate (0.4–2.2%), ethanol (0.01–2.2%), 2-phenylethanol (1.0–1.9%), (E,E)-farnesol (0.0–1.5%), beta-caryophyllene (0.5–1.2%), eugenol (0.5–1.2%), geranyl acetate (0.2–1.0%)

CAS No.: 84604-12-6 (Provence—absolute)

2-phenylethanol (64.8–73.0%), (–)-Citronellol (8.8–12.0%), alkenes (such as gamma-muurolene, alpha-pinene) and alkanes (such as tricosane, eicosane, octadecane) (1.1–8.5%), geraniol (4.9–6.4%), nerol (0.0–3.0%), eugenol (0.7–2.8%), (E,E)-farnesol (0.5–1.5%), terpinen-4-ol (0.0–1.0%), methyleugenol (0.0–0.8%)

(Tisserand and Young 2014, 405–7)

Subtle Connections: Essential Oil

Colors: Yellow *(opposite: violet),* green *(opposite: red)*

Gemstones: Citrine *(opposite: amethyst),* aventurine *(opposite: jasper)*

Chakras: Solar plexus, heart

Energy: Yin

Elements: Water, Metal

Subtle Connections: Absolute

Colors: Red *(opposite: green),* orange *(opposite: blue),* green *(opposite: red)*

Gemstones: Jasper *(opposite: aventurine),* carnelian *(opposite: aquamarine/lapis lazuli),* aventurine *(opposite: jasper)*

Chakras: Root, sacral, heart

Energy: Yin/yang

Elements: Fire

Actions and Uses

General actions: Anti-inflammatory, antiseptic, antispasmodic, antiviral, aphrodisiac, astringent, bactericidal, hydrating, skin healing, tonic

Skin: Abscesses, acne, dermatitis, dry/oily skin and scalp (balancing), eczema, herpes simplex, mature skin, shingles; makes a good toner

Respiratory system: Coughs, chronic asthma, hay fever, mouth ulcers, sore throat

Joints and muscles: Tonic to smooth muscle tissue

Circulatory system: Helps the body regulate blood pressure

Immune system: Chronic fatigue syndrome, myalgic encephalomyelitis; immune stimulant

Other: Headache/migraine, painful periods/PMS, menopausal symptoms; endocrine stimulant (hormone-like)

Associated limbic structures: Anterior thalamic nuclei, hypothalamus, amygdala, and pituitary (via the hypothalamus)

Potential psycho-emotional and spiritual support: Sedative at low dosages, stimulant at high dosages; eases agitation, anger, anxiety, depression (especially postnatal) and low mood, fear and paranoia, grief (and sense of loss), hatred, headaches (tension and hormonal), hypersensitivity, insomnia, jealousy, migraine, nervous tension, panic attacks, premenstrual tension, resentment and disappointment, sadness and despair, stress, and stress-related conditions; endocrine stimulant (hormone-like); aphrodisiac

SPIKENARD
(Nardostachys jatamansi, N. grandiflora)

Geographical location: Native to the mountains of India, and grows in the high-altitude regions of Nepal, India, and China. Biblical and Ayurvedic scriptures and other texts testify to its historical growth, production, and application in the Middle East, Europe, and India. The essential oil is distilled and produced mainly in America, Nepal, and India, with some production in Europe. Also known as muskroot. Traditionally used as a perfume, incense, and herbal sedative. Overexploitation of wild spikenard in Nepal means that cultivation of the plant is encouraged in this region.

Plant description: A tender flowering herb or plant growing up to 1 m high with pink bell-shaped flowers clustered in umbels on top of a long green stem, with dark to light green elongated or oval-shaped leaves. Related to valerian, with similar, although less pungent, odoros and sedating qualities. The roots are often traded as valerian. Ensure that your supplier obtains the essential oil from a sustainable source.

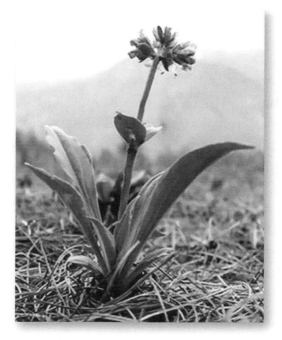

Botanical family: Valerianaceae

Extraction Method: Steam distillation of the dried, crushed rhizomes and roots

Appearance of essential oil: Deep red-orange; viscous

Odor of essential oil: Very sweet, intense, and fresh pea–like, with tones of fresh grass and slight woodiness; becomes less intense and delicately woody, with undertones of spice, fresh pea, and hay, with sweet and tenaciously lingering dry-out notes of fresh pea and hay

Compatible Serenity Essential Oils for blending: Cypress, frankincense, geranium, lavender (English and spike), patchouli, rose otto, vetivert

Safety data: Nontoxic, nonirritant, and nonsensitizing (Tisserand and Young 2014, 429)

Perfume note: Base

Principal chemical constituents: CAS No.: 8022-22-8
Nardol (10.1%), formic acid (9.4%), alpha-selinene (9.2%), dihydro-beta-ionone (7.9%), nardol isomer (4.8%), selinene isomer (type not specified) (3.9%), propionic acid (3.4%), beta-caryophyllene (3.3%),

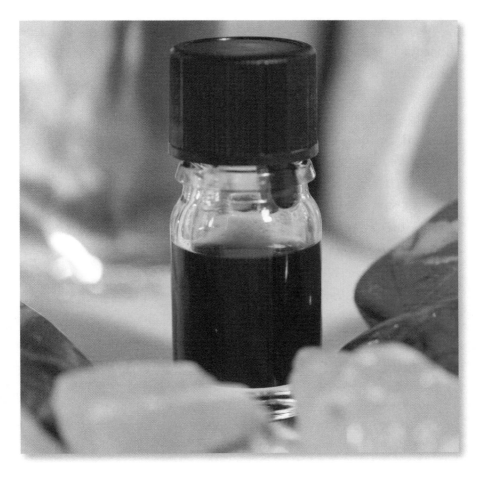

cubebol (2.9%), alpha-gurjunene (2.5%), alpha-caryophyllene (2.3%), gamma-gurjunene (2.3%), selinene isomer (type not specified) (2.2%), 7-hexadecene (2.0%), (E)-nerolidol (1.9%), calamenene (1.1%), (+)-ledene epoxy (1.0%)

(Tisserand and Young 2014, 428–29)

Subtle Connections

Colors: Red *(opposite: green)*, orange *(opposite: blue)*, green *(opposite: red)*, blue *(opposite: orange)*

Gemstones: Jasper *(opposite: aventurine)*, carnelian *(opposite: aquamarine/ lapis lazuli)*, aventurine *(opposite: jasper)*, aquamarine/lapis lazuli *(opposite: carnelian)*

Chakras: Root, sacral, heart, throat

Energy: Yang

Elements: Fire, Wood

Actions and Uses

General actions: Anti-infectious, anti-inflammatory, bactericidal, deodorant, fungicidal, rejuvenating, tonic

Skin: Inflammation, mature skin, rashes (especially when caused by nervousness)

Respiratory system: Panic attacks; calms the flow of breathing

Circulatory system: Improves circulation

Digestive system: Nervous indigestion

Other: Headache/migraine, PMS, menopausal problems

Associated limbic structures: Anterior thalamic nuclei, hypothalamus

Potential psycho-emotional and spiritual support: Balances sympathetic nervous system with parasympathetic nervous system (tonic to the sympathetic nervous system, regulates the parasympathetic nervous system); grounding; eases anxiety, grief, hatred, headaches and migraine, hyperactivity, hysteria, impatience, insomnia, irritability, menopausal symptoms, nervous indigestion, nervous tension, panic attacks, premenstrual syndrome (PMS), restlessness, stress, and stress-related conditions; sedative

TEA TREE
(Melaleuca alternifolia)

Geographical location: Native to Australia, flourishing in low-lying swampy areas in subtropical coastal regions around northeastern New South Wales and southern Queensland. Although other *Melaleuca* species are cultivated elsewhere, *M. alternifolia* does not naturally occur and is not produced outside Australia. There are six identified chemotypes of *M. alternifolia*: a terpinen-4-ol chemotype, a terpinolene chemotype, and four 1,8-cineole chemotypes. Each produces

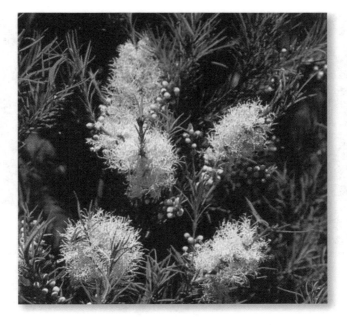

an essential oil with a distinct chemical composition, but no obvious difference has been observed to date in the bioactive capability among them. Terpinen-4-ol has antimicrobial and anti-inflammatory properties; terpinolene has antiseptic and antioxidant properties; 1,8-cineole is irritant (and this constituent is deliberately reduced in some commercial tea tree essential oils). Tea tree is also known as paperbark tree. It is usually grown from seed on commercial plantations (and harvested for distillation of the essential oil after one to three years of intense growth).

Plant description: Shrubs or small trees growing from 2 to 7 m tall, with green to dark-green ovate or lanceolate cypress-needle-like leaves. The bark is often flaky. Produces white to yellow, or greenish to pink and red, many-spiked sessile flowers with small petals on long and tightly bundled central stamens that mature to produce woody cup-shaped seed capsules, or fruits.

Botanical family: Myrtaceae

Extraction Method: Steam distillation of the leaves and terminal twigs and branches

Appearance of essential oil: Clear to pale yellow or yellow-green

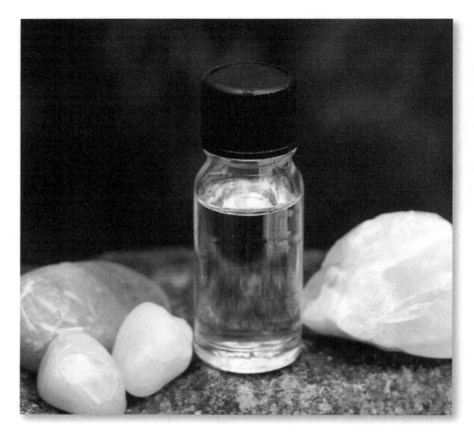

Odor of essential oil: Strongly camphoraceous, metallic tones, evolving to a warm, camphoraceous-medicinal spicy odor and finishing with little characteristic at dry out

Compatible Serenity Essential Oils for blending: Geranium, lavender (English and spike), mandarin

Safety data: Nontoxic and nonirritant; potential sensitization for some individuals

Perfume note: Top

Principal chemical constituents: CAS No.: 68647-73-4

Terpinen-4-ol (30.0–48.0%), gamma-terpinene (10.0–28.0%), 1,8-cineole (trace to15.0%), alpha-terpinene (5.0–13.0%), terpinolene (1.5–5.0%), rho-cymene (0.5–12.0%), alpha-pinene (1.0–6.0%), alpha-terpineol (1.5–8.0%), aromadendrene (trace to 7.0%), delta-cadinene (trace–8.0%), limonene (0.5–4.0%), sabinene (trace–3.5%), globulol (trace–3.0%), viridiflorol (trace–1.5%); the chemical profile is prone to altering during storage, with rho-cymene levels increasing and and alpha- and gamma-terpinene levels declining

(Carson, Hammer, and Riley 2006).

Subtle Connections

Colors: Yellow *(opposite: violet)*, green *(opposite: red)*

Gemstones: Citrine *(opposite: amethyst)*, aventurine *(opposite: jasper)*

Chakras: Solar plexus, heart

Energy: Yang

Element: Metal

Actions and Uses

General actions: Anti-infectious, anti-inflammatory, antimicrobial,* antiseptic, antiviral, bactericidal, expectorant, fungicidal, skin healing

Skin: Abscesses, acne, burns, herpes simplex, insect bites, oily skin, pimples, shingles (with geranium); cleansing

Respiratory system: Asthma, bronchitis, catarrh, colds, coughs, ear-nose-throat infections, gum disease, hay fever, mycosis, sinusitis, sore throat, tonsillitis, upper respiratory tract infections

Immune system: Chronic fatigue syndrome, myalgic encephalomyelitis; immune stimulant

Fungal infections: *Candida, Trichophyton, Epidermophyton, Malassezia,* and *Microsporum* species (ringworm, athlete's foot, et cetera; see pages 73–74)

Associated limbic structures: Anterior thalamic nuclei, hypothalamus

Potential psycho-emotional and spiritual support: Revitalizing and stimulating; cleansing; helpful for apathy, nervous exhaustion, and shock

---

*Tea tree oil is powerfully antimicrobial. It alters the permeability of invasive microbial cells, disrupting the cells' vital functions, demonstrating promising natural antibiotic potential (Vasey 2018, 93; Carson, Hammer, and Riley 2006).

VETIVERT
(Vetiveria zizanioides)

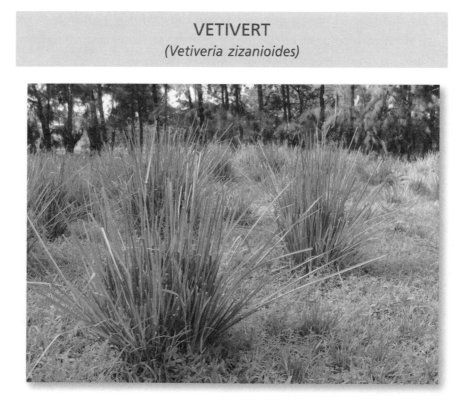

Geographical location: Native to India and widely cultivated throughout tropical regions of the world, including Haiti, Réunion, and Java. Indonesia, China, Haiti, and Java are the major producers of the essential oil, most of which, due to its remarkable enduring fixative properties, is used by the perfume industry (vetivert apparently features as an ingredient in 60 percent of all Western perfumes) (Lavania 2003). Réunion and Haiti produce a high-quality essential oil known as Bourbon vetivert, highly valued by perfumers for its roseate note. Indian vetivert (also known as khus oil) has a balsamic woody note. Other countries that produce the essential oil include Brazil, Mexico, El Salvador, and Madagascar.

Plant description: A perennial grass with tall stems and long, thin rigid leaves growing in clumps (or bunches) up to 1.5 m high and bearing brownish-purple flowers. The roots extend 2 to 4 m deep, providing good anchorage. Grown to protect soil from erosion, as fodder for

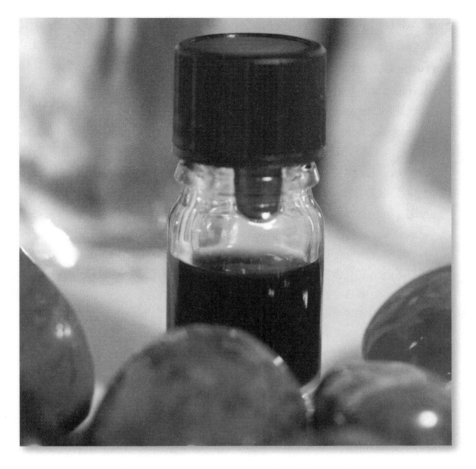

grazing animals, and to provide essential oil for perfumery, aesthetic, and medicinal purposes.

Botanical family: Poaceae (Graminae)

Extraction method: Steam distillation of the roots and rootlets (the chemical composition of the extracted essential oil is highly complex and cannot be reproduced synthetically)

Appearance of essential oil: Amber to dark brown-red; viscous

Odor of essential oil: Sweet, complex, earthy, and burnt-smoky-woody to rich, heavy, woody, earthy, and balsamic, with tenacious woody and earthy dry-out notes.

Compatible Serenity Essential Oils for blending: Frankincense, lavender (English and spike), patchouli, rose otto, spikenard

Safety data: Nontoxic and nonirritant. Generally nonsensitizing, though there have been rare reports of sensitization in hypersensitive individuals.

Perfume note: Base

Principal chemical constituents: CAS No.: 8016-96-4

Khusimol/zizanol (3.4–13.7%), vetiselinenol/isonootkatol (1.3–7.8%), cyclocopacamphan-12-ol epimer A (1.0–6.7%), alpha-cadinol (0.0–6.5%), alpha-vetivone/isonootkatone (2.5–6.4%), beta-vetivenene (0.2–5.7%), beta-eudesmol (0.0–5.2%), beta-vetivone (2.0–4.9%), khusenic acid (0.0–4.8%), beta-vetispirene (1.5–4.5%), gamma-vetivenene (0.2–4.3%), alpha-amorphene (1.5–4.1%), (E)-eudesm-4(15),7-dien-12-ol (1.7–3.7%), beta-calacorene (0.0–3.5%), gamma-cadinene (0.0–3.4%), (Z)-eudesm-6-en-11-ol (1.1–3.3%), gamma-amorphene (0.0–3.3%), ziza-5-en-12-ol (0.0–3.3%), beta-selinene (0.0–3.1%), salvia-4(14)-en-1-one (0.0–2.9%), (Z)-eudesma-6,11-diene (0.0–2.9%), khusinol (0.0–2.8%), cyclocopacamphan-12-ol epimer B (1.1–2.7%), selina-6-en-4-ol (0.0–2.7%), khusian-ol (1.5–2.6%), delta-amorphene (0.0–2.5%), 1-epi-cubenol (0.0–2.4%), khusimene/ziza-6(13)-ene (1.1–2.3%), ziza-6(13)-en-3beta-ol (0.0–2.3%), ziza-6(13)-en-3-one (0.0–2.3%), 2-epi-ziza-6(13)-en-3alpha-ol (1.0–2.2%), 12-nor-ziza-6(13)-en-2beta-ol (0.0–2.2%), alpha-vetispirene (0.0–2.2%), eremophila-1(10),7(11)-diene (0.9–2.1%), dimethyl-6,7-bicyclo-(4.4.0)-deca-10-en-one (0.0–2.0%), 10-epi-gamma-eudesmol (0.0–1.8%), alpha-calacorene (0.4–1.7%), (E)-opposita-4(15),7(11)-dien-12-ol (0.0–1.7%), prekhusenic acid (0.0–1.6%), 13-nor-eudesma-4,6-dien-11-one (0.6–1.5%), 2-epi-ziza-6(13)-en-12-al (0.0–1.5%), isovalencenol (0.0–1.5%), spirovetiva-1(10),7(11)-diene (0.0–1.5%), (E)-isovalencenal (0.7–1.4%), preziza-7(15)-ene (0.6–1.4%), (Z)-eudesma-6,11-dien-3beta-ol (0.0–1.4%), intermedeol/eudesm-11-en-4-ol (0.0–1.3%), isoeugenol (0.0–1.3%), isokhusenic acid (0.0–1.3%), elemol (0.3–1.2%), eremophila-1(10),6-dien-12-al (0.0–1.2%), juniper camphor (0.0–1.2%), khusimone (0.5–1.1%), allo-khusiol (0.0–1.1%), (E)-2-nor-zizaene (0.0–1.1%), eremophila-1(10),4(15)-dien-2-alpha-ol (0.0–1.1%), eremophila-1(10),7(11)-dien-2-beta-ol (0.0–1.1%), methyl-(E)-eremophila-1(10),7,(11)-dien-12-ether (0.0–1.1%), (Z)-isovalencenal (0.0–1.1%), funebran-15-al (0.0–1.0%), (Z)-eudesm-6-en-12-al (0.0–1.0%)

(Tisserand and Young 2014, 466)

Subtle Connections

Colors: Red *(opposite: green)*, orange *(opposite: blue)*

Gemstones: Jasper *(opposite: aventurine)*, carnelian *(opposite: aquamarine/ lapis lazuli)*

Chakras: Root, sacral

Energy: Yin

Elements: Earth, Water

Actions and Uses

General actions: Anti-arthritic, antiseptic, antispasmodic, nervous system sedative, tonic

Skin: acne, dry/oily skin, inflammation, mature skin, stimulates circulation

Respiratory system: Calms and regulates the flow of breathing (due to calming effect on the nervous system)

Joints and muscles: Aching and painful muscles, arthritis, sprains and strains

Immune system: Chronic fatigue syndrome, myalgic encephalomyelitis; immune stimulant

Fungal infections: *Candida, Epidermophyton, Microsporum,* and *Trychophyton* species (ringworm, athlete's foot, et cetera; see pages 73–74)

Other: PMS, menopausal problems

Associated limbic structures: Anterior thalamic nuclei, hypothalamus, amygdala

Potential psycho-emotional and spiritual support: Reduces symptoms of withdrawal for someone coming off medication (especially tranquilizers); eases anxiety, confusion and indecisiveness, debility, depression, hyperactivity, hypersensitivity, impatience, insomnia, menopausal symptoms, mental exhaustion, nervous tension, panic attacks, premenstrual tension, stress, and stress-related conditions; encourages feelings of tranquillity; sedative to the nervous system; grounding

7

Application

Instructions and Indications for Fifteen Methods

There are many methods of applying essential oils, and the information in this chapter will enable you to select the method most suitable to your current needs and requirements, from making a face cream to creating a therapeutic remedy or perfume.

When applied appropriately, essential oils pose little risk. However, they are best used in limited, controlled amounts, especially when they are used on a frequent basis. Citrus oils, particularly lemon, and those oils containing a high proportion of citrusy components (like pinene and limonene, which are found in pine and melissa, for example) become increasingly irritant and sensitizing as the more volatile terpene components rapidly evaporate and other components left behind transmute (for example, monoterpenes transmute into peroxides, then epoxides and alcohols); citrus oils have a short shelf life for this reason. This is an especially significant point to remember when preparing skin-care products. Thus, when you are making your own formulations using essential oils, it is very important to use high-quality, appropriately stored essential oils, to measure the essential oils carefully, to store the formulations appropriately, and to prepare them in small batches that will be used up quickly, before the essential oils have a chance to deteriorate.

For all recipes in this chapter follow the blending ratio guidelines on pages 98–99. These preparations are designed to last for a few weeks. Therefore, anticipating that your mixture will be used a little at a time, the amount of essential oil to carrier medium (cream, lotion, ointment, and so on) can be increased to its highest 5% limit: 1 drop of essential oil to 1ml of carrier medium. The blending ratio will also be determined by the type of essential oil you select. For example, chamomile (Roman and German) and rose essential oils are best used in reduced amount: their scent is very strong, and they can become irritants in high dose. Vetivert is another oil that can be used in small amounts—remember also that vetivert acts as a scent fixative and will slow the oxidation rate of other essential oils. In my experience, it is unnecessary to apply essential oils in large quantity; essential oils are still very effective applied in small amounts.

STORAGE AND SHELF LIFE

Jars, bottles, and other containers that you will use to store your formulations must be thoroughly clean and dry. Feel free to reuse glass containers as long as they are thoroughly clean and dry. Do not use plastic containers for products containing essential oils, as essential oils degrade plastic (and polystyrene).

In general, homemade products containing essential oils should be stored in a cool, dark location. They should be made in small batches that will be used up quickly. Shelf life varies depending on the particular product; the recipes in this chapter note the optimal timing. Adding antioxidant ingredients such as avocado oil, vitamin E oil, or carrot seed essential oil will slow the evaporation of the volatile components, helping to maintain the longevity of the product.

Some of the recipes in this chapter call for distilled water or hydrosols (witch hazel and rose water, for example). Hydrosols are prone to contamination, and so they (and any products made with them) have a short shelf life and must be stored appropriately (in a cool, dark place).

Safe Use: Dilution and Dosing

As noted throughout this book, essential oils should never be used neat—that is, undiluted. (Lavender and tea tree essential oils are the exceptions to this rule; they may be applied as a drop or two in first-aid situations.) The formulations described in this chapter are all a means of diluting essential oils so that they can be safely applied, whether for percutaneous (perfume, massage, cream, lotion, ointment) or direct olfactory (steam inhalation or smelling strip) absorption. Chapter 3 provides a detailed discussion of dilution and dosing. As a quick overview:

Reduced dose	1 drop of essential oil in 5 ml carrier medium = 1% blend
	1 drop of essential oil in 10 ml carrier medium = 0.5% blend
	1 drop of essential oil in 20 ml carrier medium = 0.25% blend
Normal dose	5 drops of essential oil in 10 ml carrier medium = 2.5% blend
Acute/exceptional dose	5 drops of essential oil in 5 ml carrier medium = 5% blend
Daily dose	Should not exceed 6 drops total, whether via percutaneous or direct olfactory application

CREAMS

Cream can be applied to nurture the skin, especially where it is delicate, such as the face, or in areas where it is very dry. It also makes a less slippery lubricant for deep tissue massage and baby massage.

Method

Combine the essential oil(s) of your choice with a base cream. The ratio of essential oil to base cream will depend on whether you are making face cream or body cream; see the recipes below. Use a nonperfumed, paraben-free, and preferably lanolin-free base cream. Or make your own; see the recipe on pages 244–45. Do not use base creams that contain

Applying Essential Oils: General Guidelines

1. To hone your essential oil selection, decide on your specific purpose or theme: to aid relaxation, to stimulate alertness, to create a particular ambience, to aid a particular emotion (uplifting, grounding, balancing), to aid meditation, and so on.

2. Decide whether you will use a single essential oil or a blend. A blend of essential oils offers a wider range of potential actions, but sometimes one well-chosen essential oil can be equally effective.

3. If you decide to use more than one essential oil in a blend, limit your choices to three or four essential oils and affirm their compatibility, or harmony, with one another.

4. When using more than one essential oil, aim to include different notes to enhance the balance and tenacity of your blend (remember, base-note essential oils linger longest, while top notes evaporate very quickly).

5. Avoid blending essential oils with opposite effects, like stimulating essential oils with relaxing essential oils; they will cancel each other out.

6. Avoid using the same essential oil or blend of essential oils repeatedly. Change your selection from time to time. If you are using essential oils regularly for their psycho-emotional qualities, apply reduced amounts—less is more over long periods of time. Varying the essential oils that you use will help you avoid developing a sensitivity to any particular essential oil or constituent.

7. Take breaks of abstinence. For example, use your essential oils for three or four weeks, and then have a week's break. This, too, will help prevent sensization.

8. Stop using an essential oil or blend immediately if you feel nauseous or develop a headache, skin rash, redness, or itchiness (particularly at the point of application).

9. If you are vaporizing essential oils in a communal or public area, ensure that those people sharing the space are aware that you are doing so and agree to it. Do not take for granted that everyone likes the odor of the essential oils that you like.

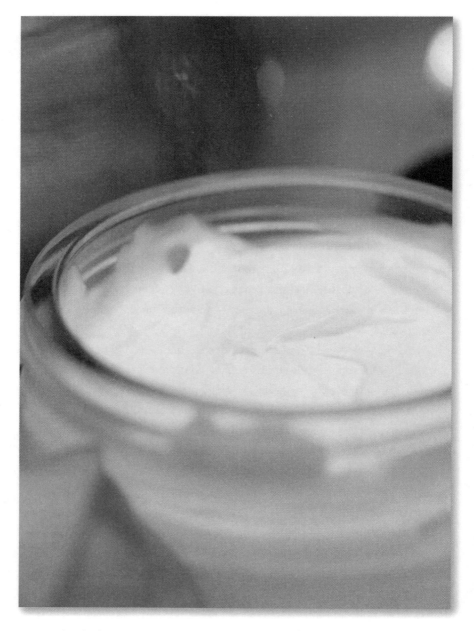

mineral oils (mineral oils do not penetrate the epidermis; instead they form a film, like an oil slick, on the skin's surface, clogging pores).

To improve the shelf life of your base cream, add an antioxidant ingredient such as vitamin E oil, avocado oil, or carrot seed essential oil, as part of your base oil or essential oil quota.

Indications

Use for:

+ Moisturizing and maintaining the suppleness of normal to dry skin
+ Alleviating cracked and chapped skin
+ Cooling and reducing redness, inflammation, and/or irritation of the skin
+ Massage lubricant for very dry skin or where a less slippery lubricant is desired

❧ Face Cream

8 drops essential oil(s) of your choice
30 grams (30 ml) base cream

1. If the cream is not already in a container with a lid, transfer it to one.
2. Make a hole in the center of the cream. Add the drops of essential oil to the hole.
3. Stir the essential oil into the cream, using a glass or wooden stirring rod, until it is evenly dispersed.
4. Tightly seal the container with its lid. Let stand for twenty-four hours in a cool, dark spot.
5. Store in a cool, dark spot and use within six weeks.

To Use

When applying the cream, it's best to remove the cream from the jar with a clean small spoon or cotton swab rather than with your fingers to avoid contamination. Replace the lid immediately after use.

❧ Body Cream

25 to 30 drops essential oil(s) of your choice
200 grams (200 ml) base cream

Prepare the body cream following the instructions for face cream (above). Store in a cool, dark spot and use within six weeks.

Creating your own homemade base cream (or lotion or ointment, pages 247–48 and 250–51) allows you to create a truly personalized remedy to meet your specific requirements. The following recipes are simple to prepare and will allow you to experiment with different combinations and consistencies.

ᕽ Homemade Base Cream

You will need small glass jars with lids (preferably amber or blue glass, although clear is fine if you will be storing your cream in the refrigerator); the number of jars required will depend on their size (e.g., 15 ml, 30 ml, 60 ml).

> **80 ml grapeseed or other appropriate plant oil(s)**
>
> **(e.g., olive, coconut, or jojoba)**
>
> **20 grams yellow beeswax**
>
> **40 ml distilled water or hydrosol of your choice (witch**
>
> **hazel, orange water, rose water, et cetera)**

1. Fill a large saucepan with a couple inches of water.
2. Set a large heatproof bowl into the saucepan. The water line should be no higher than halfway up the outside of the bowl.
3. Gently heat the water to a low simmer, ensuring that it does not bubble up and splash into the bowl.
4. Add the vegetable oil to the bowl and gently heat until it is warm (but not very hot).
5. Grate or break the beeswax into small pieces and place them in the bowl, stirring to disperse the melting wax into the warm oil. Once completely melted, remove the pan from the heat.
6. Pour the distilled water into a small saucepan and gently heat until it is warm (approximately body temperature).
7. Remove the pan from the heat, then add the distilled water, one spoonful at a time, to the warm oil and beeswax mixture, whisking each time to disperse the water evenly. Keep adding warm distilled water and whisking until your mixture has reached your desired cream-like consistency. (Once added, the water cannot be removed, so take your time and frequently check the consistency.)
8. Spoon the mixture into clean, dry jar(s) and secure the lid(s) firmly.
9. Stand the jars in very cold water to rapidly cool the mixture (the water should not rise beyond the shoulder of the jar); once cold, remove the jars and dry thoroughly.

10. Store the jars of cream in the fridge or another cool, dark place.

To Use

Do not add essential oils to your jars of homemade base cream until you are ready to use one. At that point you can open a jar and add essential oils as desired. This allows you to protect the essential oils from degrading before you are ready to use them. It also means that you can change whatever blend of essential oils you decide to add, or you can have the option of using an essential oil–free cream as a break to reduce the risk of sensitization. Unopened and stored in a cool, dark place, the jars of cream will keep for six months.

LOTIONS

A lotion is a lighter version of a cream. Like a cream, a lotion is useful for nurturing delicate, dry, and mature skin and as a less slippery alternative to massage oil.

Method

Combine the essential oil(s) of your choice with a base lotion. Use a nonperfumed, paraben-free, and preferably lanolin-free base lotion. Or you can make your own by adding distilled water and oil to a base cream; see the box on pages 247–48. Do not use base lotions that contain mineral oils (mineral oils do not penetrate the epidermis; instead they form a film, like an oil slick, on the skin's surface, clogging pores).

To improve the shelf life of your base lotion, add an antioxidant ingredient such as vitamin E oil, avocado oil, or carrot seed essential oil, as part of your base oil or essential oil quota. Note that lotion is more prone to contamination than cream due to its higher water content. You can mitigate that risk by adding antimicrobial, antifungal essential oils.

Indications

Use for:

+ Moisturizing normal, oily, and dry skin
+ Moisturizing large surface areas of skin (lotion is easier to apply compared to cream)

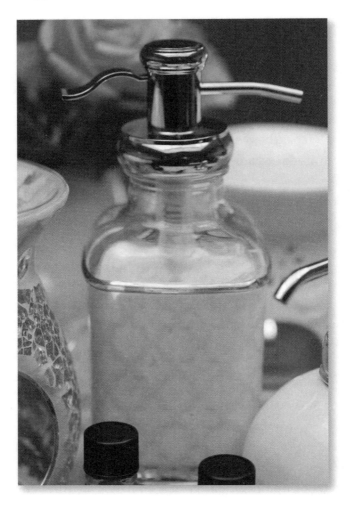

+ Moisturizing hairy skin (again, lotion is easier to apply compared to cream)
+ Massage lubricant for dry or mature skin
+ Soothing and cooling inflamed or damaged skin (watery lotions tend to evaporate quickly, which helps cool any inflammation)

❧ Lotion with Essential Oils

Using the following ratio between essential oil(s) and base lotion, you can increase the quantity of this recipe—for example, by doubling the amounts below to create 400 ml of lotion, or by adding another

12 to 15 drops of essential oil(s) and 100 ml of base lotion to create 300 ml of lotion.

25 to 30 drops essential oil(s) of your choice
200 ml base lotion

1. If the lotion is not already in a container (preferably glass or ceramic) with a lid, transfer it to one.
2. Make a hole in the center of the lotion. Add the drops of essential oil to the hole.
3. Stir the essential oil into the lotion, using a small whisk or glass or wooden stirring rod, until it is evenly dispersed.
4. Tightly seal the container with its lid. Let stand for twenty-four hours in a cool, dark spot.
5. Store in a cool, dark spot and use within six weeks.

To Use

As is the case when applying cream, it's best to remove lotion from its container without reaching into the container with your fingers to avoid contamination. Use a clean small spoon or cotton swab (replace the lid immediately after use), or use a glass or ceramic pump dispenser.

Converting Cream to Lotion

To convert cream to lotion, you simply add oil and water, alternating between the two and whisking well. Use whatever kind of oil was originally used to make the cream. If you're unsure, grapeseed and jojoba are good all-purpose oils that generally combine well with any other kinds of oils. Water added alone will reduce the consistency of your mixture. Too much base oil, however, can cause your mixture to curdle (water and oil separate when the balance between them is spoiled). You need to judge the ratio between both ingredients as you go.

Add a spoonful of the oil first, a little at a time, using a whisk to blend the oil evenly into the cream. Then add a spoonful of distilled water in the same way, using the whisk to evenly disperse the water. Keep adding oil and water, alternating and whisking well, until your lotion has reached your desired consistency. Too much vegetable oil will render your lotion very greasy.

Do not add the water and oil at the same time or your mixture may curdle; remember, your mixture may also curdle if you add too much oil. Experiment, adding the oil and water a little at a time and mixing thoroughly between additions—again, remember that you can add but not remove ingredients, so take your time.

OINTMENTS

An ointment is made like a cream but with no water. Because it is not water-based, it is less prone to contamination and has a longer shelf life, especially when essential oils are added, and it can be stored and kept on hand to use as a first-aid antiseptic salve for minor burns, stings, and insect bites.

Method

Follow the basic recipe for homemade ointment on pages 250–51, heating and combining oil and beeswax until the mixture takes on an ointment-like consistency. You can make plain ointment for uses such as lip balm or hydrating dry skin, or you can add essential oils for their antimicrobial and healing powers. To improve the shelf life of your ointment, include an antioxidant ingredient such as vitamin E oil, avocado oil, or carrot seed essential oil, as part of your base oil or essential oil quota.

Indications

Use for:

+ Antiseptic salve (minor cuts, scrapes, insect bites or stings)
+ Dry, scaly skin (apply without essential oils or as 1% blend with essential oils)
+ Lip balm (apply without essential oils)
+ Perfume pomade base (add essential oils; see chapter 4)

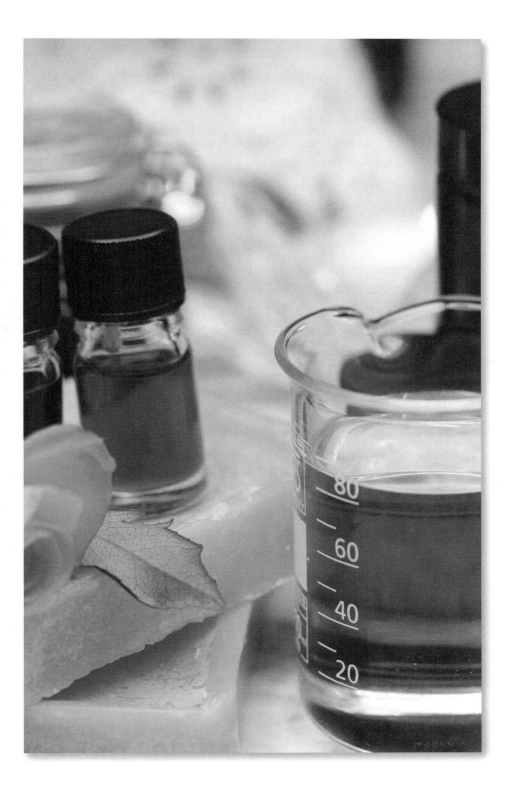

❧ Homemade Ointment

You will need five 15 ml (or g) glass jars with lids (preferably amber or blue glass, although clear glass is fine if you will be storing your ointment in the refrigerator).

> **80 ml calendula, avocado, grapeseed, or other oil**
> **20 grams yellow beeswax**
> **A cold plate or saucer for testing your mixture (place**
> **in the refrigerator for a few moments while you**
> **prepare your ingrdients)**
> **6 to 10 drops essential oil(s) of your choice (optional)**

1. Fill a large saucepan with a couple inches of water.
2. Set a large heatproof bowl into the saucepan. The water line should be no higher than halfway up the outside of the bowl.
3. Gently heat the water to a low simmer, ensuring that it does not bubble up and splash into the bowl.
4. Add the oil to the bowl and gently heat until it is warm (but not very hot).
5. Grate or break the beeswax into small pieces and place them in the bowl, stirring to disperse the melting wax into the warm oil.
6. To test the consistency of your ointment, use a clean spoon to scoop out a small amount of the mixture and drop it onto a cold plate. Allow to cool. Then test the consistency, rubbing some of the ointment onto the back of your hand to gauge. If it is too thick, gradually add more oil to the warm beeswax-oil mixture, testing each time you add more, until it reaches your desired consistency. If it is too thin, gradually add more grated beeswax.
7. When the consistency is to your liking, carefully pour the warm mixture into small glass jars.
8. Allow to cool briefly (until the ointment is just beginning to set at the edges of the jar), then divide 5 to 10 drops of your chosen essential oil(s) equally among the jars and carefully stir with a glass or wooden stirring rod to disperse them evenly throughout the mixture.
9. Secure the lids immediately, then stand the jars in very cold water (the water should not rise beyond the shoulder of the jar) to rapidly

cool the ointment and preserve the integrity of the essential oil. Once cold, remove the jars and dry thoroughly.

10. Let stand in a cool, dark place for twenty-four hours before use. Store in a cool, dark spot, where the ointment will keep for up to a year.

Antiseptic ointment: Prepare the above ointment using equal drops of lavender essential oil and tea tree essential oil, adhering to the quantities and ratios above for adding oils to the base medium.

POMADE (PERFUME OIL)

A pomade is a macerated vegetable oil—that is, an oil in which an aromatic plant has been steeped. Left to stand in warm vegetable oil (or animal fat, as the ancients used to do, a process known as enfleurage), the plant material begins to break down, surrendering its essential oil to the vegetable oil. After some time the oil is strained to remove the plant material, leaving behind an aromatic oil that has been infused with the essential oils, flavonoids (which color the infused oil), and other fat-soluble constituents from the plant. Your pomade will express a gentle nature-like fragrance, like the scent you might experience walking past flowers in a garden.

Method
Making pomade is an easy process.

❧ Homemade Pomade
Coconut oil,* jojoba oil, or grapeseed oil
Freshly picked fragrant flower heads (e.g., rose,
lavender, jasmine)—ensure that they are not wet
with dew or rain water

---

*Fractionated coconut oil is in a permanent liquid state (the long-chain fatty acids have been removed) and has a less coconutty scent. Unfractionated coconut oil is solid at room temperature or just below but becomes liquid at about 76°F. Either will work in this recipe.

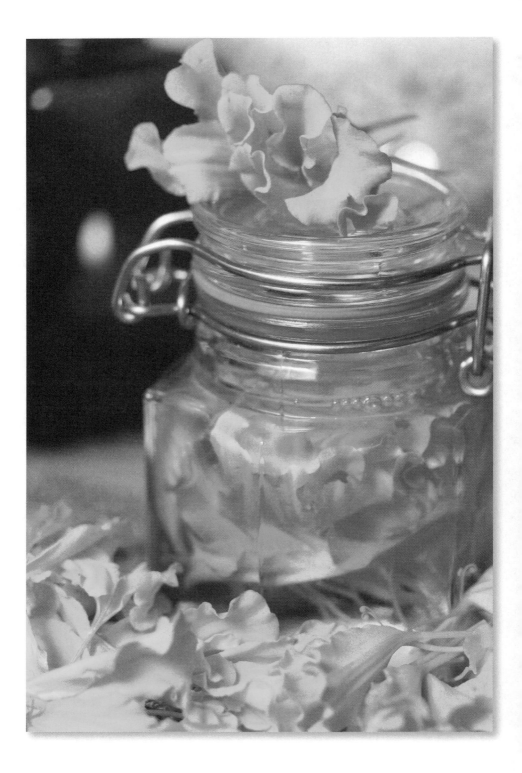

1. Fill a small jar almost to the top with the oil.
2. Add the flower heads. Stir the mixture, then seal the jar tightly with the lid.
3. Let stand for twenty-four hours.
4. Strain the flowers from the mixture. Pour the strained oil back into the jar. Discard the used flowers.
5. Repeat the above process with a fresh batch of flowers.
6. Continue to repeat the process, straining the oil and adding fresh flowers, for two to four weeks, until you feel that the oil's scent is sufficiently strong.
7. Pour the mixture into small, clean, dry bottles and seal with a lid.
8. Store the bottles in a fridge or another cool, dark place and use within one month.

To Use

Apply to your wrists, neck, or as an anointment for your feet. Wear with pleasure!

Indications

Use for:
+ Aesthetic purposes—attractant, mood, occasion, theme
+ Anxiety and depression
+ Stress and stress-related conditions

ROLLER BOTTLES

Roller bottles are best used for the application of therapeutic and aesthetic perfumes. They are convenient, safe, and easy to use.

Method

Half-fill a 10 ml roller bottle with a carrier oil, such as jojoba, borage seed, grapeseed, and so on (do not use mineral oil). Add up to 10 drops of your chosen essential oil or blend of essential oils. Top up with carrier oil to the shoulder of the bottle. Secure the roller ball cap and lid. Roll the bottle rapidly between the palms and fingers of your hands to

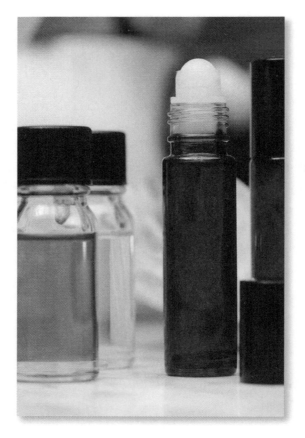

shake up and disperse the essential oils throughout the carrier oil. Let stand in a cool place for twenty-four hours to allow the essential oils to diffuse evenly into the carrier oil.

To use, remove the external cap and roll the perfume oil onto your wrists or temples as desired, replacing the lid immediately after use. Use within six weeks.

Note: The roller bottle can be reused; wash with warm soapy water, rinse, and dry thoroughly before refilling.

Indications
Use for:

+ Aesthetic purposses—attractant, mood, occasion, theme
+ Anxiety and depression
+ Headaches

✦ Improving or reinforcing memory retention

✦ Psycho-emotional moods and conditions—for example, for grief, joy, loss, nervousness, or pleasure, or to balance, calm, invigorate, sedate, or uplift

✦ Stress and stress-related conditions

NASAL INHALERS

Nasal inhalers are for therapeutic use. They are convenient and safe, even for older children, as there is no direct contact with the essential oil(s). Designed for direct personal inhalation, they are more discreet than other applications such as a perfume. Nasal inhalers offer a clean and efficient way of inhaling essential oils with immediate effect on the respiratory system (throat and lungs) and limbic system (mood,

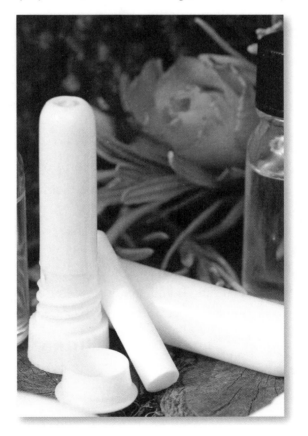

emotions, and mental clarity). They can be carried around in a pocket or bag and applied as and when required.

Method

Dismantle the nasal inhaler to remove the wadding roll inside the containing tube. Add 2 to 6 drops of your selected essential oil or blend of essential oils to the wadding roll. Replace the essential oil–infused wadding into the containing tube, secure the small base cap to seal the wadding within the tube, then screw on the protective cover.

To use, remove the cover, hold the tube to your nose, and inhale through each nostril as required. Replace the protective cover immediately after use.

Note: The plastic container can be reused; wash with warm soapy water, rinse, and dry thoroughly before reusing. Replace the wadding roll with a roll of cotton wool or tissue. Do not reuse more than two or three times.

Indications

Use for:

+ Anxiety and depression
+ Chest infections
+ Colds and flu
+ Headaches
+ Immune support (antimicrobial, anti-infectious, antiviral)
+ Improving respiration
+ Improving or reinforcing memory retention
+ Insomnia
+ Mental clarity (to clear head and thoughts)
+ Psycho-emotional moods and conditions—for example, for grief, joy, loss, nervousness, or pleasure, or to balance, calm, invigorate, sedate, or uplift
+ Sinus congestion
+ Sore throat
+ Stress and stress-related conditions

TISSUES

Tissues are a quick and easy method of therapeutic inhalation. When you add a couple drops of essential oil to a clean tissue, the essential oil molecules are able to vaporize freely with full and immediate impact and benefit. (Vaporization is limited when smelling an essential oil directly from the bottle.) This method offers a useful first-aid remedy for headaches, shock and upset, and colds and flu.

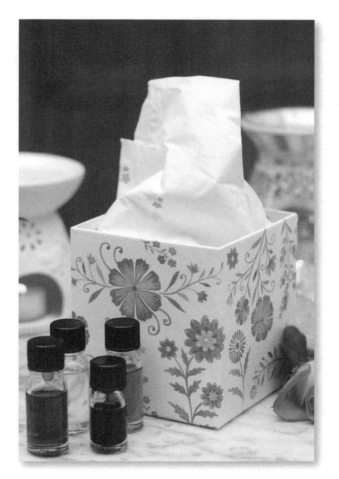

Method

Add 1 to 3 drops of your selected essential oil or blend of essential oils to the tissue. Inhale the vapors from the tissue as required. Do not allow an essential oil–infused tissue to touch the skin on your face or nose to avoid potential skin irritation.

For Immediate Need or First Aid

Here is a useful method for cases of immediate need or for first aid, such as to treat headaches, shock, and upset. Hold an essential oil–infused tissue in cupped hands, with one hand as the base and the other cupped over the palm of this hand, forming an enclosed receptacle for the tissue (thus temporarily containing the evaporating vapors), leaving a small inhaling gap between the thumb and forefinger of the upper hand. Inhale the vaporizing fragrance through the gap. Wash your hands when this exercise is finished to remove any essential oil that may have transferred from the tissue to your hands.

Indications
Use for:

+ Anxiety and depression
+ Chest infections
+ Colds and flu
+ Headaches
+ Immune support (antimicrobial, anti-infectious, antiviral)
+ Improving respiration
+ Improving or reinforcing memory retention
+ Insomnia
+ Mental clarity (to clear head and thoughts)
+ Psycho-emotional moods and conditions—for example, for grief, joy, loss, nervousness, or pleasure, or to balance, calm, invigorate, sedate, or uplift
+ Shock and upset
+ Sinus congestion
+ Sore throat
+ Stress and stress-related conditions

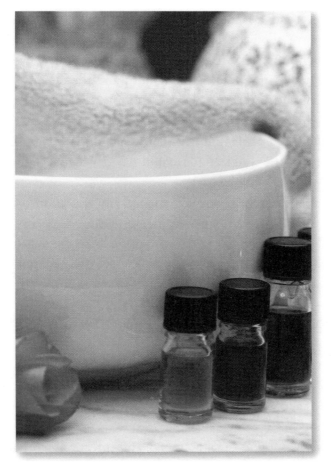

STEAM INHALATION

Another mode of therapeutic inhalation, steam is a great method for clearing the sinuses, relieving sore throats and chest infections, and decongesting the lungs. It also opens and aids the cleansing of facial pores; it is a refreshing facial sauna!

Method

You will need a kettle (or pan), water, a heat-proof bowl, tissues, essential oils, and a large towel. Before commencing, set the bowl on a stable, heat-proof surface in a safe spot away from pets and children. Heat the water in the kettle to boiling. Very carefully pour the hot water into the bowl. Allow the water to cool slightly (essential oils will vaporize too rapidly otherwise). Add 2 to 4 drops of your selected essential oil or blend of essential oils to the water.

Sit down in front of the bowl, at a height from which you can lean comfortably over it, and cover your head and the bowl with the large towel to contain the rising essential oil–infused steam vapors. Close your eyes. Breathe the vapours in through your nose and exhale through your mouth for a few minutes. Then remove the towel (come up for air). Replenish the water and essential oils if necessary and repeat the exercise two or three times.

Stop immediately if you experience any irritation or feel dizzy. Essential oils will irritate mucous membranes to a certain degree; use moderately and do not exceed the above dose. Caution must be observed and the dose reduced if the recipient has sensitivities, asthma, or epilepsy (use half the above dose—1 or 2 drops of essential oil).

Indications

Use for:

+ Anxiety and depression
+ Chest or bronchial infections or conditions
+ Colds and flu
+ Headaches
+ Immune support (antimicrobial, anti-infectious, antiviral)
+ Improving respiration
+ Insomnia
+ Loosening or encouraging the release of mucus (expectorant)
+ Mental clarity (to clear head and thoughts)
+ Psycho-emotional moods and conditions—for example, for grief, joy, loss, nervousness, or pleasure, or to balance, calm, invigorate, sedate, or uplift
+ Sinus congestion
+ Sore throat
+ Skin care: opening and cleansing pores, which helps with mitigating acne and oily skin and revitalizing facial/neck skin (rinse with cool water and/or witch hazel after steam inhalation to close pores)
+ Stress and stress-related conditions

ENVIRONMENTAL ROOM VAPORIZERS
AND DIFFUSERS

Candle-lit burners are a very popular way of diffusing essential oils and they do create a lovely ambience. However, care must be taken when using them; always ensure that the candle is extinguished before leaving the burner unattended, keep out of the reach of children, and so on.

Electric steam diffusers have improved by leaps and bounds in terms of their design and are becoming increasingly popular, especially because they are safer to use (although caution must still be applied). They tend to dispense the essential oil–infused steam more rapidly and further into the atmosphere of a room and seem to maintain the integrity of the fragrance better than other methods of diffusion.

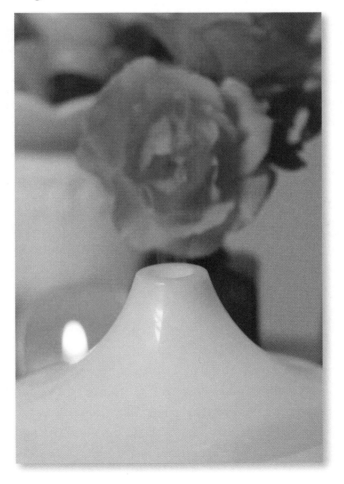

Most essential oils can be diffused in either way. However, essential oils extracted from fruits (for example, mandarin and lime), woods (for example, sandalwood, cedarwood, cypress, and pine), flowers (for example, ylang ylang, orange blossom, and of course rose) and resins (such as frankincense and myrrh), to name just a few examples, are especially refreshing, pleasant, and tenacious and can be combined to make lovely blends. Rose is one of my favorites; the otto (essential oil) is extremely expensive, but the absolute is less so and equally lovely via diffusion. Either can be purchased in a 5% blend usually mixed with jojoba oil. Both the absolute and otto are intensely perfumed, so using a very small amount is still effective.

Remember, scent preference is very personal, and what one person may really like, another person may not. When you diffuse essential oils in a communal area, be mindful that the essential oils you choose are agreeable to everyone sharing the space with you.

With environmental diffusion, our sense of smell soon becomes saturated; the brain stops acknowledging a diffuse scent after a short period of time, even though it may still be present. However, if you leave the space and then return to it, your brain should reacknowledge the scent. If it does not, this indicates that the essential oils need replenishment.

Method: Electric Fan or Steam Diffusers

These diffusers usually come with instructions regarding appropriate operation and use. Add 6 to 8 drops of an essential oil or essential oil blend, along with whatever volume of water is needed. Replenish as necessary. Rather than leaving the diffuser on constantly, use it in short bursts at chosen convenient times.

Method: Candle-Lit Diffusers

Add water to the bowl. Add 6 to 8 drops of an essential oil or essential oil blend. Light the candle. Replenish as necessary. Do not allow the water to evaporate completely; keep a small jug of water at hand to refill the diffuser. Candle-lit diffusers with deep water-holding bowls will lose water less quickly to evaporation.

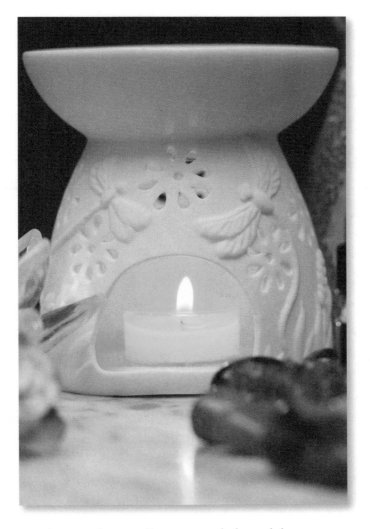

Do not leave a lit candle unattended, and be sure to set the diffuser in a spot where it cannot be knocked over or touched by children or pets.

Indications

Use for:

+ Aesthetic (environmental) perfume
+ Anxiety and depression
+ Calming
+ Improving or supporting mood

+ Improving or creating a particular ambience or theme
+ Insomnia
+ Masking unpleasant odors
+ Reducing or combating airborne microbes
+ Reducing restlessness and agitation (calming, improving mood)
+ Stress and stress-related conditions
+ Uplifting

Serenity Essential Oils to Combat Infection

Serenity Essential Oils possess powerful antimicrobial and immune-stimulant and supportive qualities. These oils may be diffused environmentally to combat or reduce, to an extent, airborne microbes and fungal spores to reduce the spread of infections. Essential oils are most effective at reducing airborne pathogens during the initial thirty minutes or so of diffusion, after which their strength diminishes as the terpenes and more active top notes disappear. To maximize this effect, keep all windows and doors closed during diffusion.

Colds and flu are caused by viruses, which tend to spread by contact and are more appropriately combated via direct inhalation and other methods of contact absorption, in conjunction with the diffusion of antimicrobial essential oils.

All of the Serenity Essential Oils offer immune-system support, but the ones listed below are immune *stimulants;* they boost and stimulate the immune system by inducing activation or increasing activity of its components.

Serenity Essential Oil Immune Stimulants

Top Notes	Middle Notes	Base Notes
Cajeput	Carrot seed	Frankincense
Mandarin, green	Chamomile, German	Patchouli
Petitgrain	Cypress	Rose otto
Tea tree	Geranium	
	Lavender, spike	

RESIN BURNERS

Resin is collected from incisions made in the bark or stem of a tree or plant and then dried. It can be heated to release the essential oil contained within. Frankincense, galbanum, and myrrh are examples of resins.

Terra-cotta and ceramic resin burners do not conduct heat as rapidly as metal ones and so are preferable in terms of safe handling, but they must be placed in a safe, stable spot where they cannot be knocked over or touched by children or pets. Metal resin burners (used, for example, in religious ceremonies) provide ornate cage-like containers, which allow the essential oil–infused smoke to permeate through holes in the structure, and are suspended on a chain so the container can safely be handled or moved once the resin is heated.

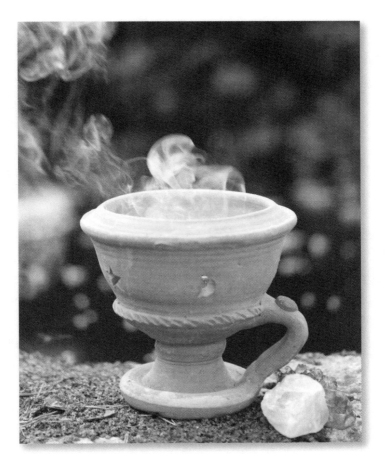

Method

Hold a small, flat piece of charcoal with long-handled pincers or twee-zers. Use a lighter or a match to light it; once the charcoal sparks, it will rapidly heat. Still using the tweezers, place the burning charcoal within the bowl of the burner and set a small piece of resin on top of it. As the charcoal heats the resin, the resin will begin to smoke as it melts and disintegrates; the essential oil is carried within the smoke that diffuses into the surrounding atmosphere.

Do not leave the resin burner unattended once it is lit. Always ensure that the charcoal and resin have burned out once you are finished with them; douse them with water if there is any doubt about whether they are extinguished.

Indications

Use for:

+ Aesthetics
+ Improving or supporting mood
+ Improving or creating a particular ambience or theme
+ Masking unpleasant odours
+ Meditation

BATHS

Essential oils can be used in the bath for therapeutic purposes as well as for relaxation. In a bath, essential oils are usually absorbed via inhalation of fragrance-infused steam, rather than via the skin. Although wetting and soaking the skin with warm water may assist percutaneous absorption, hot or warm baths tend to encourage perspiration (excretion) rather than absorption. Water, like essential oils, is drying to the skin; dispensing the essential oils in an oily carrier medium before adding them to the bathwater helps form a barrier on the skin that may prevent essential oil irritation and reduce the drying effect of water.

Method

Fill bath with water, then, just before getting in, add 6 to 8 drops of essential oil or an essential oil blend dispersed in 20 ml of vegetable oil.

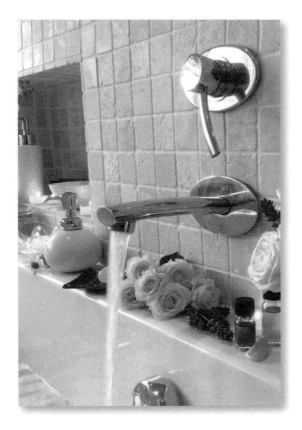

Do not use essential oils neat in the bath (water and heat exacerbate the drying and potential irritant effect of essential oils). When dispensing essential oils in vegetable oil into the bath, particularly for children, the frail, or the very elderly, be mindful that vegetable oil will render the bathtub slippery. Add the essential oils in reduced quantity for children and the elderly. Do not leave children unattended in a bath. To maximize the aromatic benefit, close the bathroom windows and doors.

The following essential oils should *not* be used in the bath because they carry a high risk of skin irritation: basil, cinnamon, citrus (any), clove, and thyme. Also avoid peppermint essential oil, which can rapidly reduce body temperature, causing excessive shivering, even hypothermia, and unpleasant sensations such as tingling and burning, particularly in sensitive areas of the body. Tea tree essential oil can also cause this cold, tingling, and burning sensation if applied to sensitive areas of the body during bathing or showering. Use vegetable oil to dilute and remove peppermint or tea tree essential oil from your skin; water intensifies the reaction.

Indications

Use for:

+ Anxiety and depression
+ Calming restlessness and agitation
+ Improving mood
+ Insomnia (bathing before bedtime)
+ Relaxation
+ Respiratory conditions, including colds and flu
+ Stress and stress-related conditions
+ Superficial skin conditions
+ Uplifting

COMPRESSES

Essential oils can be used in compresses for therapeutic applications. Compresses may be applied hot or cold. Generally speaking:

+ **Heat** releases and moves; it aids muscle relaxation and is useful for chronic conditions.
+ **Cold** constricts and reduces; it decreases blood flow and is useful for reducing heat and swelling associated with inflammation.
+ **Alternating hot and cold** is useful for exercise-induced muscle pain.

Method

To make a compress, all you need is a bowl filled with hot or cold water (depending on whether you want a warm or cold compress), a piece of absorbent material (such as flannel or a hand towel), and possibly a bandage or sheet of plastic wrap if you will want to wrap up the compress to hold it in place.

Select essential oils according to your desired outcome—for instance, to relieve pain, relax muscles, or reduce inflammation and swelling. Useful oils for aches and pains include cypress, lavender (English or

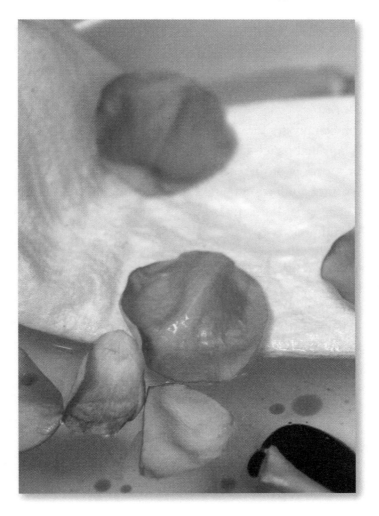

spike), chamomile (German), and galbanum as well as black pepper and marjoram. Avoid known irritant essential oils, such as basil, cinnamon, citrus, clove, and thyme, and do not use peppermint to reduce inflammation. Add about 6 drops essential oil(s) per 200 ml, or 1 cup, of water.

Soak the absorbent compress material in the essential oil and water solution. Wring it out gently; you want it to be saturated but not dripping. Apply to the affected area; wrap it with a bandage or plastic (or other waterproof) wrap if you need to secure it. Replace the compress as needed to maintain the cold or warm temperature and leave in place for twenty to thirty minutes. If alternating between warm and cold, change every five minutes, continuing for thirty to forty minutes. In the case of swelling due to muscle or ligament damage, continue until the swelling and/or pain begins to subside. Do not use hot or warm compresses in areas where there may be infection.

Indications

Use warm compresses for:

+ Abdominal issues—for example, irritable bowel syndrome (IBS), constipation, or diarrhea
+ Assisting absorption of essential oils through the skin to soft tissue and organs directly below the surface
+ Painful periods

Use cold compresses for:

+ Bruises
+ Fever
+ Headaches
+ Inflammation and swelling
+ Muscle aches and pains
+ Rheumatic or arthritic pain
+ Sprains

Use alternating hot and cold compresses for:

+ Chronic or long-term pain in a localized area
+ Exercise-induced muscle pain

GARGLES AND MOUTHWASH

Most of us are familiar with using gargles or mouthwash to freshen our breath, but when they are made with essential oils, they can also be of use therapeutically for sore throats, oral infections, and so on.

Method

Select an essential oil or two with antiseptic or anti-infectious properties; geranium, lavender, myrrh, sandalwood, or tea tree would be a good choice. Add 2 drops of essential oil to half a glass of warm water and stir to disperse the essential oils evenly.

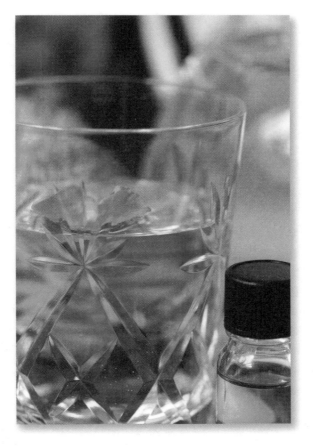

Gargle with the mixture, then spit it out. (Do *not* swallow! Essential oils can irritate the mucous lining of the digestive system unless dispensed appropriately in an emollient solution.)

Repeat twice a day, or every two hours for acute conditions, until symptoms subside (seek medical advice if symptoms persist).

Indications
Use for:
+ General oral hygiene
+ Gum infections
+ Healing after dental surgery
+ Hoarseness or loss of voice
+ Mouth ulcers
+ Oral candida

+ Pain and inflammation in the mouth
+ Respiratory problems
+ Sore throat

CLAY FACE MASKS

Clay masks are easy to make and provide wonderful healing, cleansing, and tonifying qualities for the skin. The chart on the facing page provides an overview of the qualities of different kinds of clays; use it to select the clay that is most appropriate for your needs.

You can make a very simple yet effective mask with just clay, water, and a drop of essential oil, or you can add other ingredients to extend the benefits. For example, ground rice, ground almonds, jojoba beads, or bamboo powder add exfoliating qualities. Jojoba beads are exfoliating but gentle, and they are biodegradable. Bamboo powder is exfoliating and has natural antioxidant and anti-inflammatory properties.

Other beneficial additions include vegetable oils, mashed fruits, cucumber, and even yogurt, which provide revitalizing, moisturizing, and toning qualities. Experiment with your ingredients. Have fun!

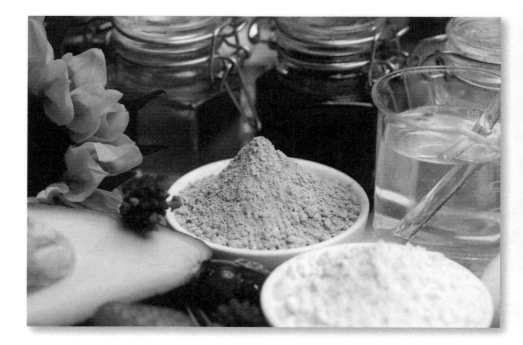

CLAYS SUITABLE FOR FACE MASKS

CLAY	USE FOR	BENEFITS	CONTENT
Green clay	Oily or acned skin	Reduces sebum production. Draws out and absorbs excess oil. Exfoliates dead skin cells. Anti-inflammatory. Skin healing.	Iron oxide, potassium, calcium, magnesium, zinc, manganese, molybdenum, and selenium
White clay	All skin types, including sensitive skin	Balances sebum production. Cleanses and tones. Anti-inflammatory. Softens the skin without dehydrating. Improves elasticity.	Pure aluminium oxide, traces of zinc, and silicon Note: White clay is sometimes called kaolin. It is generally more gentle than green clay.
Yellow clay	Devitalized, damaged, or dry/dehydrated skin	Exfoliates, tightens pores, rejuvenates tired, stressed skin. Astringent. Improves blood circulation.	Potassium, titanium, calcium, iron, aluminium, magnesium, sodium, silicon, kaolinite, mica, illite, quartz, montmorillonite, hematite, and ilmenite
Red clay	Normal to dry skin; mature skin	Improves elasticity and circulation. Rejuvenating. Anti-aging. Firms and tones the skin.	Silicon, iron, calcium, phosphorus, aluminum, sodium, titanium, magnesium, potassium, copper, smectite, quartz, illite, and kaolinite
Pink clay	Dry, sensitive skin; mature skin	Soothing, cleansing, hydrating. Exfoliates dead skin cells. Improves circulation. Restores skin vitality, elasticity, and firmness. Softens and tones skin.	Titanium, zinc, aluminum, silicon, smectite, quartz, illite, and kaolinite

Indications

Use for:

+ Balancing combination (oily and dry) skin
+ Cleansing, soothing, and hydrating the skin
+ Drawing out impurities that naturally build up within surface tissues
+ Reducing inflammation
+ Refining the appearance of pores (reduces their size)
+ Removing dead skin cells, dirt, and oil from surface tissues
+ Revitalizing the complexion

❧ Basic Face Mask

This basic recipe is ideal for cleansing and refreshing tired skin.

2 tablespoons clay powder (select the type most appropriate for you)

1 to 2 teaspoons distilled water or hydrosol (rose water, lavender hydrosol, or witch hazel, for example)*

1 drop skin-revitalizing essential oil (lavender, chamomile, rose, or geranium, for example)

1. Combine the ingredients in a glass bowl. Use a glass rod or wooden spatula to mix the ingredients until they form a smooth paste.
2. Apply immediately, using your fingertips to spread the paste evenly over your face (cheeks, forehead, chin, and neck). Leave on for about ten minutes.
3. When the mask begins to dry, it's time to remove it. (Do not allow the mask to completely dry to avoid dehydrating the skin.) Use a damp facecloth to gently wipe off any excess clay, and then rinse your face thoroughly in tepid water. Pat your face dry with a clean towel.

---

*Hydrosols are distilled; they complement the skin's natural pH balance, are less drying, and do not contain chlorine, iodine, or fluoride, which are often found in tap water. Filtered tap water can be used; distilled water, though, is preferable.

❦ Gentle Exfoliating Mask

2 tablespoons clay powder (select the type most
appropriate for you)

1 teaspoon ground almonds, ground rice, jojoba
beads, or bamboo powder

1 teaspoon oil (such as jojoba, grapeseed, or borage,
depending on your skin's needs; see the chart on
pages 56–59)

1 to 2 teaspoons hydrosol

1 drop essential oil of your choice

Prepare and apply following the instructions for the basic face mask
on the facing page.

❦ Clay Mask for Acne and Inflamed Skin

1 teaspoon green clay

1 to 2 teaspoons witch hazel

1 teaspoon ground oats

1 drop tea tree essential oil

Prepare and apply following the instructions for the basic face mask
on the facing page.

❦ Clay Mask for Oily Skin

1 teaspoon green clay

1 teaspoon jojoba oil

1 drop petitgrain essential oil

A few drops of orange floral water

Prepare and apply following the instructions for the basic face mask
on the facing page.

SELF-MASSAGE

Self-massage is a wonderful way to nurture yourself. Any movement and
stimulation of soft tissue improves circulation and lymphatic drainage.

Rhythmic movements and gentle pressure also aid muscle relaxation. Touch is also comforting.

Self-massage can be done after a bath or shower, when your skin is warm, clean, and hydrated, using lotion or vegetable oil as a lubricating medium. Add essential oils to your lotion or oil to instill further benefits.

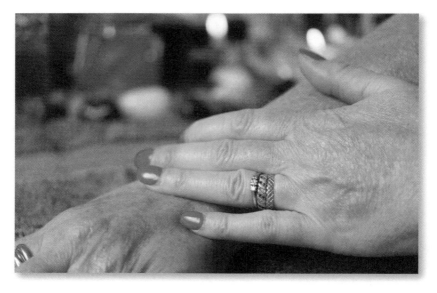

Method

Add 4 to 6 drops of your selected essential oil or essential oil blend to your chosen carrier medium, which should be contained in a small a dish or pouring jug. Place the containing vessel on a small saucer to catch drips and spills.

Pour a small amount of the oil mixture into the palm of your hand, then stroke (effleurage) the oil over the area to be massaged.

With the flat of your hand (palms, fingers, and thumbs), apply firm rhythmic stroking and circular movements to your limbs, abdomen, buttocks, shoulders, neck, and face. Gently pick up and squeeze your skin and soft tissue (the fleshy-muscled areas of your body, such as the upper arms, legs, thighs, and buttocks), again using a rhythmic motion.

Working from the feet to the head tends to be stimulating and thus is a good method for morning massage. Working from the head to the feet can be sedating and relaxing and is better suited to evening time. Do not massage over bruises, cuts, or damaged skin.

Indications

Use for:

+ Alertness (in the morning) and restfulness (in the evening)
+ Alleviating stress and stress-related conditions
+ Relaxation
+ Calming
+ Lubricating, softening, and moisturizing the skin
+ Self-empowerment
+ Soothing
+ Stimulating and improving the circulatory and lymphatic system
+ Stimulating the endocrine glands and the release of hormones
+ Stimulating the nervous system via nerve endings in the skin
+ Supporting and improving the immune system
+ Supporting detoxification via the epidermis
+ Supporting feelings of value, self-worth, and self-esteem
+ Uplifting

Massage for a Partner

Massage is a nurturing process for both the giver and the receiver. As with self-massage, apply a series of flowing rhythmic movements focusing on areas of muscle and soft tissue to improve suppleness and circulation. Start with the back, then the back of the legs, the front of the legs, the feet, the arms, and finally the head, face (forehead and cheeks), neck, and shoulders. Do not apply excessive pressure over bony areas, such as the scapula (shoulder blade) or the "floating ribs" at the base of the rib cage, over the kidney area, or over joints, especially the back of the knees, the elbows, and the wrists. Of course, a simple back massage is also very effective, as is a head, neck and shoulder massage, or hand or foot massage.

Conclusion

You can buy ready-made essential oil formulas from most essential oil suppliers, and you can find many, many recipes for formulas online or in books—including this one! But in my experience, the effectiveness of an essential oil or an essential oil blend depends entirely on whether or not it is appropriate for the user. As we've discussed, essential oils have multidynamic properties and wide-ranging dynamics, and they trigger uniquely individualized responses in each of us. For this reason, ready-made formulas are useful as guides while you are learning about essential oils, or as a "quick fix" first-aid remedy for an emergency, but they do not represent a truly holistic therapy. For this, you need knowledge and experience. I hope that this book will have given you a touch of the former; I encourage you to go out and gain as much of the latter as you can. Experience—a willingness to explore, try, and learn—is key!

Remedies are far more effective when the recipient proactively participates in essential oil selection. The recipient is able to tap into their own subtle needs and healing dynamics, consciously or unconsciously, which will influence their choice (through attraction to, acceptance of, or rejection of an essential oil) and thus optimize their holistic self-healing capacity. So, as well as perusing this book and all the information it contains, use your own sense of smell. Apply this sense as a portal to delve into your inner self. Follow your feelings, allowing this sense to instinctively and intuitively guide you to what your body, mind, and spirit truly need.

Essential oils are wonderful tools in this respect, as they appear to naturally awaken intuitive processes. What is your signature condition, or your reason for using essential oils? What outcome do you wish to achieve? Select oils that complement your purpose, then follow your nose. Become the creative, inquisitive traveler; enjoy your sensory journey and find the innate healer within *you*.

Appendix

Adverse Reaction
Report Form

It is useful to keep a log of any adverse event, small or large. This information should be stored in a database for reference—at the very least, your own, and/or ideally one organized by a related professional body. The example below provides a guide.

ADVERSE REACTION REPORT (ARR)

Name:	Date:
Address:	Tel: Mobile: E-mail:
Database agency address:	Tel: Mobile: E-mail:

Any information submitted will be treated in complete confidence. However, details of essential oil(s) and the nature of the reaction reported will be kept on a universal Essential Oil Safety Database for general reference.

1	Essential Oil		ml/drop
	Common name:	Latin name:	
	Batch number:	Supplier:	
	Essential Oil Blend (if appropriate)		ml/drop
	Common name:	Latin name:	
	Batch number:	Supplier:	
	Common name:	Latin name:	
	Batch number:	Supplier:	
	Common name:	Latin name:	
	Batch number:	Supplier:	
	Common name:	Latin name:	
	Batch number:	Supplier:	

2	Carrier Medium		ml		ml
	Vegetable oil (1):			Vegetable oil (2):	

Cream		Lotion		Gel		Clay		Other	

Details:

Blend ratio:	1%	2%	5%	Other %	Number of drops or ml		Quantity of carrier medium	ml/gm

3	Method of Application / Use

Inhalation: steam or tissue	Perfume: therapeutic/ aesthetic	Topical: face cream, body lotion, etc.	Topical first aid ointment, neat, etc.	Local compress area_____	
Massage (local)	Area of body:	Massage (full body)	Room vaporizer	Other:	

Details (including frequency of use, e.g., three times a day, once a day, once a week, etc.)

4	Details of Person Affected				
	Female		Male		Age	Occupation

	Number of applications prior to reaction		Details
	Reason for use / application / treatment	Details	
	Known / identified allergies or sensitivities (e.g. hay fever, peanuts, pet fur, etc.)	Details	
	Known / identified skin conditions (e.g. eczema, dermatitis, psoriasis, dry, etc.)	Details	

5	Details of Other Treatments	
	G.P. treatment (or other healthcare professional treatment) applied concurrently with essential oil, aromatherapy use or treatment	Details
	Medication prescribed / taken concurrently with essential oil, aromatherapy use or treatment	Details
	Other treatment applied concurrently with essential oils, aromatherapy use or treatment (e.g. dietary supplements, homeopathy, acupuncture, herbalism, reflexology, massage)	Details

6	Description of the Nature of the Adverse Reaction				
	Allergy		Sensitivity		Irritation	
	Details (including treatment of reaction)				

Bibliography

Alexander, M. 2001a. "Aromatherapy and Immunity: How the Use of Essential Oil Aids Immune Potentiality in Four Parts. Part 1: How Essential Oil Odourants Affect Immune Potentiality." *International Journal of Aromatherapy* 11, no. 2: 63–66.

Alexander, M. 2001b. "Aromatherapy and Immunity: How the Use of Essential Oils Aid Immune Potentiality. Part 2: Mood-Immune Correlations, Stress and Susceptibility to Illness and How Essential Oil Odorants Raise This Threshold." *International Journal of Aromatherapy* 11, no. 3: 152–66.

Armstrong, F., and V. Heidingsfeld. 2001. "Aromatherapy for Deaf and Deaf-Blind People Living in Residential Accommodation." *International Journal of Aromatherapy* 11, no. 1: 26–34.

Australian Tea Tree Industry Association (ATTIA). 2006. "Growing Tea Trees." Article on the ATTIA website.

Balazs, T. 1999. "The Fragrant Brain." *International Journal of Aromatherapy* 9, no. 2: 57–61.

Balazs, T., and R. Tisserand. 1999. "German Chamomile." *International Journal of Aromatherapy* 9, no. 1: 15–21.

Ballabh, P., A. Braun, and M. Nedergaard. 2004. "The Blood-Brain Barrier: An Overview. Structure, Regulation, and Clinical Implications." *Neurobiology of Disease* 16, no. 1: 1–13.

Ballard, C. G., J. T. O'Brian, K. Reichelt, and E. K. Perry. 2002. "Aromatherapy as a Safe and Effective Treatment for the Management of Agitation in Severe Dementia: The Results of a Double-Blind, Placebo-Controlled Trial with Melissa." *Journal of Clinical Psychiatry* 63, no. 7: 553–58.

Battaglia, Salvatore 2003. *The Complete Guide to Aromatherapy,* 2nd ed. Brisbane, Australia: International Centre of Holistic Aromatherapy.

Becker, Todd. 2012. "Hormesis and the Limbic System." Published January 2, 2012, on the Getting Stronger website.

Bensafi, M. 2012. "The Role of the Piriform Cortex in Human Olfactory Perception: Insights from Functional Neuroimaging Studies." *Chemosensory Perception* 5, no. 1: 4–10.

Bensouilah, J. 2002. "Aetiology and Management of Acne Vulgaris. *International Journal of Aromatherapy* 12, no. 2: 99–104.

———. 2003. "Psoriasis and Aromatherapy." *International Journal of Aromatherapy* 13, no. 1: 2–8.

Bensouilah, J., and P. Buck. 2006. *Aromadermatology: Aromatherapy in the Treatment and Care of Common Skin Conditions.* Oxon, U.K.: Radcliffe Publishing.

Benveniste, B., and N. Azzo. 1992. "Geranium Oil." *Technicolour Bulletin and Newsletter* 11, July 1 (Kato Worldwide Ltd., Mount Vernon, NY). Found in Tisserand, R., and R. Young, *Essential Oil Safety,* 2nd ed. (London: Churchill Livingstone, 2014), 293.

Berkowsky, B. 2001. "The Soul Nature of Rose Oil." *International Journal of Aromatherapy* 11, no. 1: 35–39.

Beshara, M. C., and D. Giddings. 2002. "Use of Plant Essential Oils in Treating Agitation in a Dementia Unit: 10 Case Studies." *International Journal of Aromatherapy* 12, no. 4: 207–12.

Boelens, M. H., and H. Boelens. 1997. "Differences in Chemical and Sensory Properties of Orange Flower Oil and Rose Oils Obtained from Hydrodistillation and from Superficial CO_2 Extraction." *Perfumer and Flavorist* 22, 31–35. Found in Tisserand, R., and R. Young, *Essential Oil Safety,* 2nd ed. (London: Churchill Livingstone, 2014), 405.

Boskabady, M. H., M. N. Shafei, Z. Saberia, and S. Amini. 2011. "Pharmacological Effects of *Rosa damascena.*" *Iranian Journal of Basic Medical Sciences* 14, no. 4: 295–307.

Bourke, J., I. Coulson, and J. English. 2009. "Guidelines for the Management of Contact Dermatitis: An Update." *British Journal of Dermatology* 160, no. 5: 946–54.

Broughan, C. 1999. "Fragrant Mechanisms." *International Journal of Aromatherapy* 9, no. 4: 166–67.

———. 2000. "Cultural Influences on Fragrance Perception." *International Journal of Aromatherapy* 10, no. 1 & 2: 54–61.

———. 2002. "Odours, Emotions, and Cognition: How Odours May Affect Cognitive Performance." *International Journal of Aromatherapy* 12, no. 2: 92–98.

Bruns, K. 1978. "Ein Beitrag zur Untersuchang unf Qualitatsbewertung von Patchouliol." *Parfumerie Kosmetik* 59: 109–15. Found in Tisserand, R., and R. Young, *Essential Oil Safety,* 2nd ed. (London: Churchill Livingstone, 2014), 382.

Buchbaur, G., L. Jirovetz, W. Jagar, C. Plank, and H. Dietrich. 1993. "Fragrance Compounds and Essential Oils with Sedative Effects upon Inhalation." *Journal of Pharmaceutical Sciences* 82, no. 6: 660–64.

Buckle, J. 2007. *Clinical Aromatherapy,* 2nd ed. London: Churchill Livingstone.

Burfield, T. 2002. "Odour Profiling (of Essential Oils) and Subjectivity." Synopsis of a lecture given at the RQA's 12th Anniversary Conference at

Regent's College Conference Center, London, March 9, 2002. Available on Tony Burfield's Magazine Page online.

———. 2003. "The Adulteration of Essential Oils—and the Consequences to Aromatherapy & Natural Perfumery Practice." Presentation to the International Federation of Aromatherapists Annual AGM, London. October 11, 2003. Transcript available on Tony Burfield's Aroma Pages website.

———. 2010. "Is Excessive Regulation Destroying the Perfumery Art?" Presentation to the British Society of Perfumers. March 2010. Transcript available on the Anya's Garden Natural Perfumes website.

Burns, A., E. Perry, C. Holmes, P. Francis, J. Morris, M. J. Howes, P. Chazot, G. Lees, and C. Ballard. 2011. "A Double-Blind Placebo-Controlled Randomized Trial of *Melissa officinalis* Oil and Donepezil for the Treatment of Agitation in Alzheimer's Disease." *Dementia and Geriatric Cognitive Disorders* 31, no. 2: 158–64.

Bushdid, C., M. O. Magnasco, L. B. Vosshall, and A. Keller. 2014. "Humans Can Discriminate More Than 1 Trillion Olfactory Stimuli." *Science* 343, no. 6177: 1370–72.

Busse, D., P. Kudella, N.-M. Gruning, et al. 2014. "A Synthetic Sandalwood Odorant Induces Wound Healing Process in Human Keratinocytes via Olfactory Receptor OR2AT4." *Journal of Investigative Dermatology* 134: 2823–32.

Caelli, M., J. Porteous, C. F. Carson, R. Heller, and T. V. Riley. 2001. "Tea Tree Oil as an Alternative Topical Decolonisation Agent for Methicillin-Resistant Staphylococcus Aureus." *International Journal of Aromatherapy* 11, no. 2: 97–99.

Cal, K. 2006. "Skin Penetration of Terpene from Essential Oils and Topical Vehicles." *Planta Medica* 72, no. 4: 311–16.

Carlson, N. R. 2013. *Physiology of Behavior,* 11th ed. Boston: Pearson.

Carpentieri-Rodrigues, L. N., J. M. Zanluchi, and I. H. Grebogi. 2007. "Percutaneous Absorption Enhancers: Mechanisms and Potential." *Brazilian Archives of Biology and Technology* 50, no. 6: 949–61.

Carson, C. F., K. A. Hammer, and T. V. Riley. 2006. "*Melaleuca alternifolia* (Tea Tree) Oil: A Review of Antimicrobial and Other Medicinal Properties." *Clinical Microbiology Reviews* 19, no. 1: 50–62.

Chevallier, A. 2001. *Encyclopedia of Medicinal Plants.* London: Dorling Kindersley.

Chialva, F., G. Gabri, P. A. P. Liddle, and F. Ulian. 1982. "Qualitative Evaluation of Aromatic Herbs by Direct Headspace GC Analysis." *Journal of High Resolution Chromatography* 5, no. 4: 182–88. Found in Tisserand, R., and R. Young, *Essential Oil Safety,* 2nd ed. (London: Churchill Livingstone, 2014), 244.

Child, N. D., and E. E. Benarroch. 2013. "Anterior Nucleus of the Thalamus: Functional Organization and Clinical Implications." *Neurology* 81, no. 21: 1869–76.

Clarke, Sue. 2002. *Essential Chemistry for Safe Aromatherapy.* London: Churchill Livingstone.

Complementary and Natural Healthcare Council (CNHC). n.d. "What Is Aromatherapy." CNHC website. Accessed June 10, 2019.

Damian, Peter, and Kate Damian. 1995. *Aromatherapy: Scent and Psyche: Using Essential Oils for Physical and Emotional Well-Being.* Rochester, Vt.: Healing Arts Press.

Davidson, J. L. 2002. "Aromatherapy and Work-Related Stress." *International Journal of Aromatherapy* 12, no. 3: 145–51.

Deans, S. G., and K. P. Svoboda. 1988. "Antibacterial Activity of French Tarragon (*Artemisia dracunculus* Linn.) Essential Oil and Its Constituents During Ontogeny." *Journal of Horticultural Science and Biotechnology* 63, no. 3: 503–8.

de Vries, E. H., J. Kuiper, A. G. de Boer, T. J. C. Van Berkel, and D. D. Breimer. 1997. "The Blood-Brain Barrier in Neuroinflammatory Diseases." *Pharmacological Reviews* 49, no. 2: 143–56.

Duke, Jim. 1998. "Fragrant Planet Aromathematics." *International Journal of Aromatherapy* 9, no. 1: 22–35.

Durell, S. 2002. "An Aromatherapy Service for People with a Learning Disability." *International Journal of Aromatherapy* 12, no. 3: 152–56.

Elemento Minerals. n.d. "Our Clays" (a breakdown of clays and mineral components). Elemento Minerals website. Accessed 2014.

European Chemicals Agency (ECHA). n.d. "Essential Oils." Accessed on ECHA website, June 14, 2019.

Forbes, R. M., A. R. Cooper, and H. H. Mitchel. 1953. "The Composition of the Adult Human Body as Determined by Chemical Analysis." *Journal of Biological Chemistry* 203: 359–66.

Francis, G. W., and Y. T. H. Bui. 2015. "Changes in the Composition of Aromatherapeutic Citrus Oils during Evaporation." *Journal of Evidence-Based Alternative and Complementary Medicine* 421695.

Friedmann, T. S. 2009. "Attention Deficit and Hyperactive Disorder (ADHD)." *International Journal of Clinical Aromatherapy* 6, no. 2: 33–36.

Fujiwara, R., T. Komori, and M. Yokoyama. 2002. "Psychoneuroimmunological Benefits of Aromatherapy." *International Journal of Aromatherapy* 12, no. 2: 72–82.

Gattefossé, Rene-Maurice. 1937. *Gattefosse's Aromatherapy.* Reprint 1995. Saffron Walden, U.K.: C. W. Daniel.

Gerber, Richard. 2001. *Vibrational Medicine: The #1 Handbook of Subtle-Energy Therapies.* Rochester, Vt.: Bear & Co.

Ghannadi, A., and S. Amree. 2002. "Volatile Constituents of *Ferula gummosa* Boiss. from Kashan, Iran." *Journal of Essential Oil Research* 14: 420-21. Found in Tisserand, R., and R. Young, *Essential Oil Safety,* 2nd ed. (London: Churchill Livingstone, 2014), 290.

Gienger, Michael. 2004. *Crystal Power, Crystal Healing: The Complete Handbook.* London: Cassell Illustrated.

Gilbert, A. N., S. C. Knasko, and J. Sabini. 1997. "Sex Differences in Task

Performance Associated with Attention to Ambient Odor." *Archives of Environmental and Occupational Health* 57: 195–99.

Gimble, Theo. 1994. *Healing with Colour and Light.* London: Gaia Books.

———. 2002. *The Colour Therapy Workbook: The Classic Guide from the Pioneering Paperback.* London: Gaia Books.

———. 2005. *The Healing Energies of Colour.* London: Gaia Books.

Godfrey, H. 2006a. "Carers Aroma Wellness: Post Course Report." *Aromatherapy Times* 1, no. 71: 22–25.

———. 2006b. "Evaluation of Complementary and Alternative Medicine." *Aromatherapy Times* 1, no. 68: 13–15.

———. 2007. "Case Work Supervision in Context." *Aromatherapy Times* 1, no. 74: 15–17.

———. 2009a. "Essential Oils: Complementary Treatment for Attention Deficit Hyperactive Disorder." *International Journal of Clinical Aromatherapy* 6, no. 1: 14–22.

———. 2009b. "The Evaluation of CAM in Routine Practice." *Aromatherapy Times* 1, no. 71: 22–25.

———. 2011. *Essential Oil Technician Pilot Course 2009–2010: Reflective Overview of Process and Outcome of Course.* End of Module Report, University of Salford, Greater Manchester (unpublished).

Grieve, M. 1931. "Galbanum." In *A Modern Herbal.* Available on the Botanical. com website.

Griffin, C. A., K. A. Kafadar, and G. K. Pavlath. 2009. "MOR23 Promotes Muscle Regeneration and Regulates Cell Adhesion and Migration." *Developmental Cell* 17, no. 5: 649–61.

Guba, R. 1999. "Wound Healing: A Pilot Study Using an Essential Oil–Based Cream to Heal Dermal Wounds and Ulcers." *International Journal of Aromatherapy* 9, no. 2: 67–74.

Haze, S., K. Sakai, and Y. Gozu. 2002. "Effects of Fragrance Inhalation on Sympathetic Activity of Normal Adults." *Japanese Journal of Pharmacology* 90, no. 3: 247–53.

Herz, R. 2016. "The Role of Odor-Evoked Memory in Psychological and Physiological Health." *Brain Sciences* 6, no. 3: 22.

Herz, R., and G. C. Cupchick. 1995. "The Emotional Distinctiveness of Odor-Evoked Memories." *Chemical Senses* 20, no. 5: 517–28.

Herz, R., C. McCall, and L. Cahill. 1999. "Hemispheric Lateralization in the Processing of Odor Pleasantness versus Odor Names." *Chemical Senses* 24, no. 6: 691–95.

Holmes, C., V. Hopkins, C. Hensford, et al. 2002. "Lavender Oil as a Treatment for Agitated Behavior in Severe Dementia: A Placebo Controlled Study." *International Journal of Geriatric Psychiatry* 17, no. 4: 305–8.

Holmes, P. 1999a. "Frankincense Oil: The Rainbow Bridge." *International Journal of Aromatherapy* 9, no. 4: 156–61.

———. 1999b. "Uplifting Oils: The Treatment of Depression in Clinical

Aromatherapy." *International Journal of Aromatherapy* 9, no. 3: 102–4.

Hummel, A. E., and A. Livermore. 2002. "Intranasal Chemosensory Function of the Trigeminal Nerve and Aspects of Its Relation to Olfaction. *International Archives of Occupational & Environmental Health* 75, no. 5: 305–13.

Ilmberger, J., E. Heuberger, C. Mahrhofer, et al. 2001. "The Influence of Essential Oils on Human Attention: 1. Alertness." *Chemical Senses* 26, no. 3: 239–45.

Jager, W., G. Buchbbauber, L. Jirovetz, H. Dietrich, and C. Plank. 1992. "Evidence of the Sedative Effect of Neroli Oil, Citronella and Phenylethyl Acetate on Mice." *Journal of Essential Oil Research* 4, no. 4: 387–94.

Jelinek, A., and B. Novakova. 2001. "The Psychotherapeutic Use of Essential Oils." *International Journal of Aromatherapy* 11, no. 2: 100–102.

Jellinek, J. S. 1997. "Psychodynamic Odor Effects and Their Mechanisms." *Cosmetics and Toiletries* 112, no. 9: 61–72.

———. 1999. "Odours and Mental States." *International Journal of Aromatherapy* 9, no. 3: 115–20.

Jirovetz, L., G. Buchbauer, W. Jager, et al. 1992. "Analysis of Fragrance Compounds in Blood Samples of Mice by Gas Chromatography, Mass Spectrometry with Chemical Ionization and Selected Ion Monitoring." *Biology and Mass Spectrometry* 20: 801–3. Found in Tisserand, R., and R. Young, *Essential Oil Safety,* 2nd ed. (London: Churchill Livingstone, 2014), 405.

Joels, M. 2008. "Functional Actions of Corticosteroids in the Hippocampus." *European Journal of Pharmacology* 583, no. 2–3: 312–21.

Jung, C. G. 1971. *Psychological Types.* Vol. 6 of *Collected Works of C. G. Jung,* 3rd ed. Princeton, N.J.: Princeton University Press.

Keller, A., and L. A. Vosshall. 2004. "Human Olfactory Psychophysics. *Current Biology* 14, no. 20: R875–78.

Kerr, J. 2002. "The Use of Essential Oils in Healing Wounds." *International Journal of Aromatherapy* 12, no. 4: 202–6.

Kirk-Smith, M. 2003. "The Psychological Effects of Lavender I: In Literature and Plays." *International Journal of Aromatherapy* 13, no. 1: 18–22.

Knecht, S., B. Dräger, M. Deppe, et al. 2000. "Handedness and Hemispheric Language Dominance in Healthy Humans." *Brain: A Journal of Neurology* 123, 12: 2512–18.

Kovar, K. A., B. Gropper, and D. Friess. 1987. "Blood Levels of 1,8-cineole and Locomotor Activity of Mice after Inhalation and Oral Administration of Rosemary Oil." *Planta Medica* 53: 315–18.

Kovats, E. 1987. "Composition of Essential Oils Part 7: Bulgarian Oil of Rose (*Rosa demascena* Mill)." *Journal of Chromatography* 406: 185–222. Found in Tisserand, R., and R. Young, *Essential Oil Safety,* 2nd ed. (London: Churchill Livingstone, 2014), 404.

Koyama, Y., H. Babdo, F. Yamashita, et al. 2012. "Comparative Analysis of Percutaneous Absorption Enhancement by D-limonene and Oleic Acid Based on a Skin Diffusion Model." *Journal of Advanced Pharmaceutcial Technology & Research* 3, no. 4: 216–23.

Kringelbach, M. L. 2005. "The Orbitofrontal Cortex: Linking Reward to Hedonic Experience." *Nature Reviews Neuroscience* 6: 691–702.

Kusmirek, Jan. 2002. *Liquid Sunshine: Vegetable Oils for Aromatherapy.* Glastonbury, England: Floramicus.

Kyle, L. 1999. "Aromatherapy for Elder Care." *International Journal of Aromatherapy* 9, no. 4: 170–77.

Lavania, Umesh. 2003. "Other Uses, and Utilization of Vetiver: Vetiver Oil." University of Lucknow (January).

Lawless, Julia. 1995. *The Illustrated Encyclopedia of Essential Oils: The Complete Guide to the Use of Oils in Aromatherapy and Herbalism.* Shaftesbury, Dorset, U.K.: Element.

Lawrence, B. M. 1979. *Essential Oils 1976–1978.* Wheaton, Ill.: Allured Publishing. Found in Tisserand, R., and R. Young, *Essential Oil Safety,* 2nd ed. (London: Churchill Livingstone, 2014).

———. 1989. *Essential Oils 1981–1987: Patchouli.* Wheaton, Ill.: Allured Publishing, 15. Found in Tisserand, R., and R. Young, *Essential Oil Safety,* 2nd ed. (London: Churchill Livingstone, 2014), 382.

———. 1993. *Essential Oils 1988–1991: Galbanum, Petitgrain.* Wheaton, Ill.: Allured Publishing, 82–83, 107–11. Found in Tisserand, R., and R. Young, *Essential Oil Safety,* 2nd ed. (London: Churchill Livingstone, 2014), 290, 375.

———. 1995a. *Essential Oils 1988–1991.* Wheaton, Ill.: Allured Publishing. Found in Tisserand, R., and R. Young, *Essential Oil Safety,* 2nd ed. (London: Churchill Livingstone, 2014), 5.

———. 1995b. "Progress in Essential Oils: Cypress." *Perfumer and Flavorist* 20: 34. Found in Tisserand, R., and R. Young, *Essential Oil Safety,* 2nd ed. (London: Churchill Livingstone, 2014), 265.

———. 1996. "Progress in Essential Oils: Mandarin." *Perfumer and Flavorist* 21: 25–28. Found in Tisserand, R., and R. Young, *Essential Oil Safety,* 2nd ed. (London: Churchill Livingstone, 2014), 342.

———. 1998. "Progress in Essential Oils: Chamomile Roman." *Perfumer and Flavorist* 6: 49. Found in Tisserand, R., and R. Young, *Essential Oil Safety,* 2nd ed. (London: Churchill Livingstone, 2014), 244.

Lee, John. 1998. *The Crystal and Mineral Guide: An Uncomplicated Journey through the A-Z of Crystals.* Baldoyle, Ireland: Aeon Press.

Leffingwell, John C. 2002. "Olfaction—Update No. 5." *Leffingwell Reports* 2, no. 1.

———. n.d. "Olfaction: A Review." On the website of Leffingwell and Associates. Accessed 2014.

Lemme, P. 2009. "The Use of Essential Oils in Psychiatric Medication Withdrawal." *International Journal of Clinical Aromatherapy* 6, no. 2: 15–23.

Lockie, Andrew. 1998. *The Family Guide to Homeopathy: The Safe Form of Medicine for the Future.* London: Hamish Hamilton.

Lu, T., F. Gasper, R. Marriot, et al. 2007. "Extraction of Borage Seed Oil by Compressed CO_2: Effect of Extraction Parameters and Modelling." *Journal of Supercritical Fluids* 41, no. 1: 68–73.

Ludvigson, H. W., and T. R. Rottman. 1989. "Effects of Ambient Odors of Lavender and Cloves on Cognition, Memory, Affect and Mood." *Chemical Senses* 14: 525–36.

Mahalwal, V. S., and M. Ali. 2002. "Volatile Constituents of the Rhizomes of *Nardostachy jatamansi* DC. *Journal of Essential Oil Bearing Plants* 5: 83–89. Found in Tisserand, R., and R. Young, *Essential Oil Safety,* 2nd ed. (London: Churchill Livingstone, 2014), 429.

Marolfi, M., M. Sirousfard, and A. Ghanadi. 2015. "Evaluation of the Effect of Aromatherapy with *Rosa damascena* Mill. on Hospitalized Children in Selected Hospitals Affiliated to Isfahan University of Medical Sciences in 2013." *Iranian Journal of Nursing and Midwifery Research* 20, no. 2: 247–54.

Maury, M. 1995. *Marguerite Maury's Guide to Aromatherapy: The Secret of Life and Youth—A Modern Alchemy.* Saffron Walden, U.K.: C. W. Daniel.

Mazzoni, V., F. Tomi, and J. Casanova. 1999. "A Daucane-type Sesquiterpene from *Daucus carota* Seed Oil." *Flavour and Fragrance Journal* 14, no. 5: 268–72. Found in Tisserand, R., and R. Young, *Essential Oil Safety,* 2nd ed. (London: Churchill Livingstone, 2014), 233.

Milchard, M. J., R. Clery, N. DeCosta, et al. 2004. "Application of Gas-Liquid Chromatography to the Analysis of Essential Oils." *Perfumer and Flavorist* 29: 28–36. Found in Tisserand, R., and R. Young, *Essential Oil Safety,* 2nd ed. (London: Churchill Livingstone, 2014), 224, 382.

Miniga, J., and J. E. Thoppil. 2002. "Studies on Essential Oil Composition and Microbicidal Activities of Two South Indian Species." *International Journal of Aromatherapy* 12, no. 4: 213–15.

Miyake, J., M. Nakagawa, and Y. Asakura. 1991. "Effects of Odours on Humans: Effects on Sleep Latency." *Chemical Senses* 16, no. 1: 184.

Miyazaki, Y., S. Takeuchi, M. Yatagai, and S. Kobayashi. 1991. "The Effect of Essential Oils on Mood in Humans." *Chemical Senses* 16, no. 1: 183.

Moss, M., and L. Oliver. 2014. "Plasma 1,8-cineole Correlates with Cognitive Performance Following Exposure to Rosemary Essential Oil Aroma." *Therapeutic Advances in Psychopharmacology* 2, no. 3: 103–13.

Motl, O., J. Hodacova, and K. Ubik. 1990. "Composition of Vietnamese Cajeput Essential Oil." *Flavour and Fragrance Journal* 5: 39–42. Found in Tisserand, R., and R. Young, *Essential Oil Safety,* 2nd ed. (London: Churchill Livingstone, 2014), 224.

Moyjay, G. 1996. *Aromatherapy for Healing the Spirit: A Guide to Restoring Emotional and Mental Balance through Essential Oils.* London: Gaia Books Limited.

Murray, M. A. n.d. "Our Chemical Senses: Olfaction." Teacher resource developed as part of the "Neuroscience for Kids" program maintained on the website of the University of Washington.

Mycology Online. "Trichophyton." Entry on the Mycology Online website hosted by the University of Adelaide, Australia.

National Center for Complementary and Integrative Health (NCCIH). 2019. "Aromatherapy with Essential Oils (PDQ)—Patient Version." Last updated May 21, 2019. National Institutes of Health website.

Nazzaro, Filomena, Florinda Fratianni, Raffaele Coppola, and Vincenzo De Feo. 2017. "Essential Oils and Antifungal Activity." *Pharmaceuticals (Basel)* 10, no. 4: 86.

NHR Organic Oils. 2015. "Safety Data Sheet: Organic Mandarin Essential Oil – Green *(Citrus reticulata)*." Brighton, UK.

Ni, X., M. M. Suhail, Q. Yang, et al. 2012. "Frankincense Essential Oil Prepared from Hydrodistillation of *Boswellia sacra* Gum Resins Induces Human Pancreatic Cancer Cell Death in Cultures and in a Xenograft Murine Model." *BMC Complementary and Alternative Medicine* 12: 253.

Norfolk Essential Oils. 2017. "Safety Data Sheet: Lavender Oil." 12/09/2017. Pates Farm, Wisbech, England.

Okabe, H., K. Takayama, A. Ogura, and T. Nagai. 2006. "Effect of Limonene and Related Compounds on the Percutaneous Absorption of Indomethacin." *Planta Medica* 72, no. 4.

Oschman, James. n.d. *The Living Matrix Connective Tissue Concept.* Available on the website of the Insitute of Bioenergetic & Informational Healthcare.

Patil, Kiran. 2019. "Properties of Coconut Oil." Organic Facts website. Last updated February 19, 2019.

Pauli, A. 2001. "Antimicrobial Properties of Essential Oil Constituents." *International Journal of Aromatherapy* 11, no. 3: 126–33.

Pengelly, A., J. Snow, S. Y. Mills, et al. 2012. "Short-Term Study on the Effects of Rosemary on Cognitive Function in an Elderly Population." *Journal of Medicinal Food* 15, no. 1: 10–17.

Perry, E. 2006. "Aromatherapy for the Treatment of Alzheimer's Disease." *Journal of Quality Research in Dementia,* 3.

Pitman, V. 2000. "Aromatherapy and Children with Learning Difficulties." *Aromatherapy Today* 15: 20–23.

Pluznick, J. L., D.-J. Zou, X. Zhang, et al. 2008. "Functional Expression of the Olfactory Signaling System in the Kidney." *Proceedings of the National Academy of Science* 106, no. 6: 2059–64.

Prasanthi, D., and P. K. Lakshmi. 2012. "Terpenes: Effect of Lipophilicity in Enhancing Transdermal Delivery of Alfuzosin Hydrochloride." *Journal of Advanced Pharmaceutical Technology & Research* 3, no. 4: 216–23.

Pulsifer, M. B., J. Brandt, C. F. Salorio, et al. 2004. "The Cognitive Outcome of Hemispherectomy in 71 Children." *Epilepsia* 45, no. 3: 243–54.

Rana, V. S., J. P. Juyal, and M. A. Blazquez. 2002. "Chemical Constituents of Essential Oil of *Pelargonium graveolens* Leaves." *International Journal of Aromatherapy* 12, no. 4: 216–18.

Romeo, R. D., R. Bellani, L. N. Karatsoreos, et al. 2005. "Stress History and

Pubertal Development Interact to Shape Hypothalamic-Pituitary-Adrenal Axis Plasticity." *Endocrinology* 147, no. 4: 1664–74.

Ryan, S. 2004. *Vital Practice—Stories from the Healing Arts: The Homeopathic and Supervisory Way*. Portland, Dorset, U.K.: Sea Change.

Sabir, A., A. Unver, and Z. Kara. 2012. "The Fatty Acid and Tocopherol Constituents of the Seed Oil Extracted from 21 Grape Varieties (*Vitis* spp.)." *Journal of the Science of Food and Agriculture* 92, no. 9: 1982–87.

Saeki, Y., and M. Shiohara. 2001. "Physiological Effects of Inhaling Fragrances." *International Journal of Aromatherapy* 11, no. 3: 118–33.

Salvo, Susan G. 2003. *Massage Therapy Principles and Practice,* 2nd ed. Philadelphia: W. B. Saunders.

Sarasto, H. 2001. "Treatment of an Elderly Asthma Sufferer with Aromatherapy (a Case History)." *International Journal of Aromatherapy* 11, no. 2: 103–7.

Sawamura, M., U. S. Son, H. S. Choi, et al. 2004. "Compositional Changes in Commercial Lemon Essential Oils for Aromatherapy." *International Journal of Aromatherapy* 14, no. 1: 27–36.

Schierling, R. 2012. "Fascia Transmits Messages Acting as Second Nervous System." Published July 12, 2012, on the Dr. Russell Schierling website.

Schmidt, E. 2003. "The Characteristics of Lavender Oils from Eastern Europe." *Perfumer and Flavorist* 28: 48–60. Found in Tisserand, R., and R. Young, *Essential Oil Safety,* 2nd ed. (London: Churchill Livingstone, 2014), 326.

Schnaubelt, Kurt 1995. *Advanced Aromatherapy: The Science of Essential Oil Therapy*. Rochester, Vt.: Healing Arts Press.

———. 1999. *Medical Aromatherapy: Healing with Essential Oils*. Berkeley, Calif.: North Atlantic Books.

Schwienbacher, I., M. Fendt, R. Richardson, and H. U. Schnitzler. 2004. "Temporary Inactivation of the Nucleus Accumbens Disrupts Acquisition and Expression of Fear-Potentiated Startle in Rats." *Brain Research* 1027, no. 1–2: 87–93.

Scientific Committee on Consumer Products (SCCP). 2005. "Opinion on Furocoumarins in Cosmetic Products." SCCP/0942/05. Found in Tisserand, R., and R. Young, *Essential Oil Safety,* 2nd ed. (London: Churchill Livingstone, 2014), 326.

Sheppard-Hanger, Sylla. 1995. *The Aromatherapy Practitioner Reference Manual*. Tampa, Fla.: Atlantic Institute of Aromatherapy.

Singh, B., R. Kumar, S. Bhandari, et al. 2007. "Volatile Constituents of Natural *Boswellia serrata,* Oleo-Gum-Resin and Commercial Samples." *Flavour and Fragrance Journal* 22: 145–47. Found in Tisserand, R., and R. Young, *Essential Oil Safety,* 2nd ed. (London: Churchill Livingstone, 2014), 288.

Sorensen, J. 2001. *The Hormonal Activity of* Vitex agnus castus *and Its Importance in Therapy*. Prepublished lecture paper (forwarded by the author).

Southwell, L. A., and I. A. Stiff. 1995. "Chemical Composition of an Australian Geranium Oil." *Journal of Essential Oil Research* 7: 545–47. Found in

Tisserand, R., and R. Young, *Essential Oil Safety,* 2nd ed. (London: Churchill Livingstone, 2014), 293.

Spehr, M., G. Gisselmann, A. Poplawski, et al. 2003. "Indentification of a Testicular Odorant Receptor Mediating Human Sperm Chemotaxis." *Science* 299, no. 5615: 2054–58.

Srinivas, S. R. 1986. "Atlas of Essential Oils." New York: Self-published. Found in Tisserand, R., and R. Young, *Essential Oil Safety,* 2nd ed. (London: Churchill Livingstone, 2014), 244.

Stangor, Charles. 2012. *Beginning Psychology.* Chapter 4, "Sensing and Perceiving." Available online from Andy Schmitz, 2012 Book Archive.

Stone, A. 2014. "Smell Turns Up in Unexpected Places." *New York Times,* October 13, 2014.

Stone, H., B. Williams, and J. A. Carregal. 1968. "The Role of the Trigeminal Nerve in Olfaction." *Experimental Neurology* 21, no. 1: 11–19.

Sullivan, T. E., B. K. Schefft, J. S. Warm, et al. 1995. "Recent Advances in the Neuropsychology of Human Olfaction and Anosmia." *Brain Injury* 9, no. 6: 641–46.

Svoboda, K. P., A. N. Karavia, and V. McFarlane. 2001. "Case Study: The Effects of Selected Essential Oils on Mood, Concentration and Sleep in a Group of 10 Students Monitored for 5 Weeks." *International Journal of Aromatherapy* 12, no. 3: 157–61.

Swanson, L. W. 2000. "Cerebral Hemisphere Regulation of Motivated Behavior." *Brain Research* 886: 113–164.

Tisserand, Robert. 1997. *The Art of Aromatherapy.* Saffron Walden, U.K.: C. W. Daniel.

———. 2012. "Rosemary Boosts Brain Power!" An article on the Robert Tisserand website, posted March 1, 2012.

———. 2015. "Frankincense Essential Oil and Cancer: Why EOs and Chemotherapy Don't Always Mix." A question-and-answer on the Robert Tisserand website, published March 26, 2015.

———. n.d. "Definition." Definition of aromatherapy on Robert Tisserand website, accessed June 14, 2019.

Tisserand, Robert, and Tony Balacs. 1995. *Essential Oil Safety: A Guide for Health Professionals.* London: Churchill Livingstone.

Tisserand, Robert, and Rodney Young. 2014. *Essential Oil Safety,* 2nd ed. London: Churchill Livingstone.

Toga, A. W., and P. M. Thompson. 2003. "Mapping Brain Asymmetry." *Nature Reviews Neuroscience* 4, no. 1: 37–48.

Tsutsulova, A. L., and R. A. Antonova. 1984. "Analysis of Bulgarian Daisy Oil." *Maslo-Zhirovaya Promyshlennost* 11: 23–24. Found in Tisserand, R., and R. Young, *Essential Oil Safety,* 2nd ed. (London: Churchill Livingstone, 2014), 242.

Tucker, A. O., and M. J. Maciarello. 1988. "Nomenclature and Chemistry of the Kazanlik Damask Rose and Some Potential Alternatives from the

Horticultural Trade of North America and Europe." In Lawrence, B. M., B. D. Mookherjee, and B. J. Willis, eds., *Flavours and Fragrances: A World Perspective* (Amsterdam: Elsevier), 99–114. Found in Tisserand, R., and R. Young, *Essential Oil Safety,* 2nd ed., (London: Churchill Livingstone, 2014), 405.

Valnet, Jean. 1980. *The Practice of Aromatherapy.* Reprint 1996. Saffron Walden, U.K.: C. W. Daniel.

Vann S., and J. Aggleton. 2004. "The Mammillary Bodies: Two Memory Systems in One?" *Nature Reviews Neuroscience* 5, no. 1: 35–44.

Vasey, Christopher. 2018. *Natural Antibiotics and Antivirals: 18 Infection-Fighting Herbs and Essential Oils.* Rochester, Vt.: Healing Arts Press.

Volz, K. G., R. Rübsamen, and D. Y. von Cramon. 2008. "Cortical Regions Activated by the Subjective Sense of Perceptual Coherence of Environmental Sounds: A Proposal for a Neuroscience of Intuition." *Cognitive Affective & Behavioral Neuroscience* 8, no. 3: 318–28.

Ward, A. M., A. P. Shultz, W. Huiibers, K. R. Van Diik, T. Heddon, and R. A. Sperling. 2014. "The Parahippocampal Gyrus Links the Default-Mode Cortical Network with the Medial Temporal Lobe Memory System." *Human Brain Mapping* 35, no. 3: 1061–73.

Watts, Martin. 2000. *Essential Oil Safety Data.* Churchill, Oxfordshire: Medical Aromatherapy Training Services; Essentially Oils Limited.

Whichello Brown, Denise. 1996. *Teach Yourself Aromatherapy.* London: Hodder Headline.

Wildwood, Chrissie. 1996. *Bloomsbury Encyclopaedia of Aromatherapy.* London: Bloomsbury.

———. 1997. *The Complete Guide to Reducing Stress.* London: Piatkus.

Williams, David G. 2006. *The Chemistry of Essential Oils: An Introduction for Aromatherapists, Beauticians, Retailers and Students.* Weymouth, Dorset: Michelle.

Wills, Pauline. 1992. *The Reflexology and Colour Therapy Workbook.* Shaftesbury, Dorset: Element.

Wilson, Kathleen J. W., and Anne Waugh. 1998. *Anatomy and Physiology in Health and Illness.* London: Churchill Livingstone.

Worwood, Valerie Ann. 1996a. *The Fragrant Mind.* London: Doubleday.

———. 1996b. *The Fragrant Pharmacy.* London: Bantam Books.

Zani, F., G. Massimo, S. Benvenuti, et al. 1991. "Studies on the Genotoxic Properties of Essential Oils with *Bacillus subtilis* Rec-assay and Salmonella/Microsome Reversion Assay." *Planta Medica* 57: 237–41. Found in Tisserand, R., and R. Young, *Essential Oil Safety,* 2nd ed. (London: Churchill Livingstone, 2014), 244.

Index

About the Author

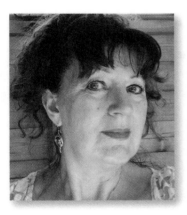

Heather studied at the University of Salford, where she was awarded a joint honors degree in counseling and complementary medicine and master's certificates in integrated mindfulness and supervision of counseling and therapeutic relationships. She also gained a postgraduate teaching certificate from Bolton Institute. She worked at the College of Health and Social Care at the University of Salford for a number of years, fulfilling multiple roles. She served as a program lead and lecturer in integrated therapy, complementary therapy, aromatherapy, communication, and professional skills.

Heather has had a number of articles and research papers published in associated professional journals, including the *International Journal of Clinical Aromatherapy* (IJCA). A fellow of the International Federation of Aromatherapists (IFA), she was chair of education in 2013 and supports the IFA's educational program in an advisory capacity and as an examiner. She is also a member of the Federation of Holistic Therapists (FHT). Through her private practice, Heather continues to provide professional training, essential oil therapy treatments, professional supervision for therapists, professional development, and introductory workshops. Visit her website at

www.aromantique.co.uk

BOOKS OF RELATED INTEREST

Essential Oils for Mindfulness and Meditation
Relax, Replenish, and Rejuvenate
by Heather Dawn Godfrey, PGCE, BSc

The Healing Intelligence of Essential Oils
The Science of Advanced Aromatherapy
by Kurt Schnaubelt, Ph.D.

Advanced Aromatherapy
The Science of Essential Oil Therapy
by Kurt Schnaubelt, Ph.D.

Essential Oils in Spiritual Practice
Working with the Chakras, Divine Archetypes,
and the Five Great Elements
by Candice Covington
Foreword by Sheila Patel, M.D.

Aromatherapy for Healing the Spirit
Restoring Emotional and Mental Balance with Essential Oils
by Gabriel Mojay

The Art of Aromatherapy
The Healing and Beautifying Properties of the Essential Oils of Flowers
and Herbs
by Robert B. Tisserand

Holistic Reflexology
Essential Oils and Crystal Massage in Reflex Zone Therapy
by Ewald Kliegel

Natural Antibiotics and Antivirals
18 Infection-Fighting Herbs and Essential Oils
by Christopher Vasey, N.D.

INNER TRADITIONS • BEAR & COMPANY
P.O. Box 388
Rochester, VT 05767
1-800-246-8648
www.InnerTraditions.com
Or contact your local bookseller

DEC - - 2019